THE ACADEMY COLLECTION
QUICK REFERENCE GUIDES FOR FAMILY PHYSICIANS

CONDITIONS OF AGING

THE ACADEMY COLLECTION
QUICK REFERENCE GUIDES FOR FAMILY PHYSICIANS

CONDITIONS OF AGING

LANYARD K. DIAL, MD
Director, Family Practice Residency
Director, Geriatric Services
Ventura County Medical Center
Associate Professor of Family Medicine
UCLA School of Medicine
Los Angeles, California

Series Medical Editor
RICHARD SADOVSKY, MD, MS

Associate Professor of Family Medicine
State University of New York Health Science Center
Brooklyn, New York

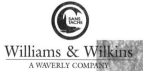

Williams & Wilkins
A WAVERLY COMPANY

BALTIMORE • PHILADELPHIA • LONDON • PARIS • BANGKOK
BUENOS AIRES • HONG KONG • MUNICH • SYDNEY • TOKYO • WROCLAW

Editor: Jonathan W. Pine, Jr.
Development Editor: Robert Newman, Co Medica, Inc
Project Manager, AAFP: Leigh McKinney
Managing Editor: Molly L. Mullen
Marketing Manager: Daniell Griffin
Project Editor: Ulita Lushnycky
Design Coordinator: Mario Fernandez

351 West Camden Street
Baltimore, Maryland 21201-2436 USA

Rose Tree Corporate Center
1400 North Providence Road
Building II, Suite 5025
Media, Pennsylvania 19063-2043 USA

Printed in the United States of America

Library of Congress Cataloging-in-Publication Data
Dial, Lanyard K.
    Conditions of aging / Lanyard K. Dial.
        p.   cm — (The Academy collection—quick reference guides for family physicians)
    "American Academy of Family Physicians."
    Includes bibliographical references and index.
    ISBN 0-683-30421-6
    1. Geriatrics—Handbooks, manuals, etc.   2. Aged—Diseases—Handbooks, manuals, etc.
3. Family medicine—Handbooks, manuals, etc.   I. American Academy of Family Physicians.
II. Title.   III. Series.
    [DNLM: 1. Geriatrics handbooks.   WT 39 D536c 1998]
RC952.55.D53   1998
618.97—dc21
DNLM/DLC   98-22643
for Library of Congress   CIP

The publishers have made every effort to trace the copyright holders for borrowed material. If they have inadvertently overlooked any, they will be pleased to make the necessary arrangements at the first opportunity.

To purchase additional copies of this book, call our customer service department at **(800) 638–0672** or fax orders to **(800) 447–8438.** For other book services, including chapter reprints and large quantity sales, ask for the Special Sales department.

Canadian customers should call **(800) 665–1148,** or fax **(800) 665–0103.** For all other calls originating outside of the United States, please call **(410) 528–4223** or fax us at **(410) 528–8550.**

Visit Williams & Wilkins on the Internet: http://www.wwilkins.com or contact our customer service department at **custserv@wwilkins.com.** Williams & Wilkins customer service representatives are available from 8:30 am to 6:00 pm, EST, Monday through Friday, for telephone access.

99 00 01 02 03
1 2 3 4 5 6 7 8 9 10

To the two greatest loves of my life,
my sweetheart and wife Mary
and my daughter Hannah.

Thanks,
Lanyard

SERIES INTRODUCTION

Family practice is a unique clinical specialty encompassing a philosophy of care rather than a modality of care provided to a specific segment of the population. This philosophy of providing longitudinal care for persons of all ages in the complete context of their physical, emotional, and social environments was modeled by general practitioners, the parents of our modern specialty. To provide this kind of care, the family physician needs a broad knowledge base, appropriate evaluation tools, effective interventions, and patient education.

The knowledge base needed by a family physician is extraordinarily large. The American Academy of Family Physicians and other organizations provide clinical education through conferences and journals. Individual family physicians have written journal articles about a specific clinical topic or have tried to cover the broad knowledge base of family medicine in a single volume. The former are helpful, but may cover only a narrow segment of medicine, while the latter may not provide the depth needed to be useful in actual patient care.

The Academy Collection: Quick Reference Guides for Family Physicians is a series of books designed to assist family physicians with the broad knowledge base unique to our specialty. The books in this series have all been written by practicing family physicians who have special interest in the topics, and the chapters have been formatted to provide easy access to information needed at varying stages in the physician-patient encounter. Each volume is unique because each author has personalized the volume and provided a unique family physician perspective.

This series is not meant to be a final reference for the family physician who seeks a comprehensive text. The series also does not cover every topic that may be encountered by the family physician. The series does offer, in a depth determined appropriate by the authors, the information needed by the physician to handle the majority of patient encounters. The series also provides information to make patient care a combined doctor-patient effort. Specific patient education materials have been included where appropriate. Readers can contact the American Academy of Family Physicians Foundation for other resources.

The topics selected for the **Academy Collection** were chosen based on what family physicians said they needed. The first group of books covers office procedures, conditions of aging, and some of the most challenging diagnoses seen in family practice. Future books in the series will address musculoskeletal problems, skin conditions, occupational/environmental medicine, children's health, and gastrointestinal problems.

I welcome your comments. Please contact me at the American Academy of Family Physicians with your suggestions (Rick Sadovsky, M.D., Series Editor, The Academy Collection, c/o AAFP, 8880 Ward Parkway, Kansas City, MO 64116; e-mail: academycollection@aafp.org). This collection is meant to be useful to you and your patients.

Richard Sadovsky, MD, MS
Series Editor

CONTENTS

Diagnostic Chart for Conditions of Aging

Clinical Manifestations	Concurrent Finding	Diagnosis Considerations
Depressed/down in dumps	Alcohol use	• Alcohol abuse
	Comorbid illness	• Organic disorder
	Death of a loved one	• Bereavement reaction
	Disturbance in normal daily activities	• Major depressive disorder (p. 43)
	Identifiable stressful event or serious medical condition	• Adjustment disorder
	Lasting 2 years or longer but not fulfilling criteria for major depression	• Dysthymia (p. 43)
	Lesser depressive symptoms associated with higher use of health care services	• Subsyndromal depression (p. 43)
	Medication use (see p. 47 for a list)	• Medication-induced depression (p. 43)
	Multiple somatic complaints	• Mood or anxiety disorder • Somatoform disorder
	Seasonal pattern	• Major depressive disorder
	"Stable instability" and intense reaction to perceived rejection	• Borderline personality disorder
	Substance/alcohol abuse or dependence	• Depression secondary to substance abuse
	Cognitive dysfunction	• Depression (p. 43) • Alzheimer's disease (p. 29) • Parkinson's disease (p. 91) • Cerebrovascular accident
	Mania	• Bipolar disorder
	Manic episodes	• Bipolar illness • Schizophrenia
Falls	Decreased hearing or vision	• Altered environmental perception
	Lightheadedness associated with standing or position changes	• Orthostatic hypotension

continued

Diagnostic Chart for Conditions of Aging *continued*

Clinical Manifestations	Concurrent Finding	Diagnosis Considerations
	Palpitations	• Arrhythmias
	History of syncope or focal neurologic findings	• CNS disorder (e.g., tumor, stroke, seizures)
	Impediments at home or in environment	• Extrinsic falls (p. 119)
	Lightheadedness, giddiness	• Presyncopal episode
	Loss of consciousness; may occur with cough, rising from bed for urination	• Syncope
	Poor diet	• Nutritional deficiency
	Precipitating medications (e.g., phenothiazines, methyldopa, many antipsychotics)	• Parkinson-like changes
	Abnormal "get up and go" test	• Gait or balance disturbance • Vertigo • Fatigue • Weakness
	Abnormal position and/or vibratory sense	• Cerebellar disorder • Neuropathy • Extrapyramidal derangement
	Diminished joint ROM	• Musculoskeletal disease
	Fever, tachycardia	• Acute illness
	Gait abnormality	• Cerebrovascular accident • Upper motor neuron disease • Parkinson's disease (p. 91) • Alcohol abuse • Multiple sclerosis • Cerebellar tumor • Normal pressure hydrocephalus • Arterial occlusion • Vitamin B_{12} deficiency • Spondylosis • Myositis

continued

Diagnostic Chart for Conditions of Aging *continued*

Clinical Manifestations	Concurrent Finding	Diagnosis Considerations
		• Polymyalgia rheumatica • Osteoarthritis (p. 77) • Foot disorder
	Hand tremor, slowness and stiffness, loss of balance, autonomic dysfunction	• Parkinson's disease (p. 91)
	Increased respiratory rate	• Congestive heart failure (CHF) (p. 1) • Pneumonia
	Joint motion leads to sensations or sound of popping or grinding	• Osteoarthritis (p. 77)
	Lower extremity weakness	• Gait or balance disturbance (p. 119)
	Motor and/or sensory function deficits	• Neurologic system disease
	Nail problems and metatarsal conditions	• Foot disabilities
	Seborrhea, sialorrhea	• Parkinson's disease (p. 91)
	Tremor at rest	• Parkinson's disease (p. 91)
	Weight loss	• Dehydration • Systemic disease • Depression (p. 43)
	Abnormal EKG	• Ischemia • Arrhythmias • CHF (p. 1)
Fatigue	Acute onset	• Viral or bacterial infections • Cardiac disease
	Behavioral changes	• Substance abuse • Anxiety disorder • Major depression (p. 43) • Meningitis • Encephalitis
	Depressed	• Major depression (p. 43) • Hypothyroidism • Dietary factors

continued

Diagnostic Chart for Conditions of Aging *continued*

Clinical Manifestations	Concurrent Finding	Diagnosis Considerations
	Dyspnea	• CHF (p. 1) • Coronary artery disease (CAD) • Chronic obstructive pulmonary disease (COPD) (p. 17)
	Irritability, breathlessness and numerous somatic complaints	• Anxiety
	Most severe in the morning	• Psychologic cause
	Multiple medications	• Polypharmacy
	Nocturia	• Benign prostatic hypertrophy (BPH) or other urethral obstruction • Urinary tract infection (UTI) • Diabetes mellitus or insipidus • CHF • Renal insufficiency • Cirrhosis with ascites
	Precipitated by psychosocial factors	• Chronic anxiety or stress
	Sleep disturbance/insomnia	• Major depression (p. 43) • Anxiety disorder • Sleep apnea
	Sleeping excessively during day	• Narcolepsy
	Swelling in ankles and around eyes	• Nephrotic syndrome
	Use of antihistamines, tranquilizers, antihypertensives	• Medicine-induced fatigue
	Coordination problems, balance problems, tremors	• Parkinson's disease (p. 91)
	Decreased breath sounds, hyper-resonance of the chest	• COPD (p. 17)
	Edema and pulmonary rales	• CHF (p. 1) • Renal insufficiency
	Enlarged heart, an S3 gallop	• CHF (p. 1)
	Fever	• Viral or bacterial infection • Rheumatologic condition • Chronic fatigue syndrome

continued

Diagnostic Chart for Conditions of Aging *continued*

Clinical Manifestations	Concurrent Finding	Diagnosis Considerations
	Fever, sore throat	• Viral syndrome • Chronic fatigue syndrome • Bacterial pharyngitis
	Focal muscle weakness	• Multiple sclerosis • Neurologic disorder • Myasthenia gravis • Myositis
	Generalized musculoskeletal aching or stiffness with specific tender sites, but normal joint/muscle exam and normal labs	• Fibromyalgia • Fibrositis
	Hearing deficit, tinnitus	• Ear disorders
	Hepatic tenderness	• Hepatitis
	Hepatosplenomegaly	• Infectious mononucleosis • Cancer
	Midsystolic click or late systolic murmur	• Mitral valve prolapse
	Resting tachycardia	• CHF (p. 1) • Arrhythmia • Anemia
	Unintended weight loss	• HIV disease • Depression • Malignancy • Dietary factors • Rheumatologic disorder • Collagen disorder • Dehydration • Systemic disease
	Wheezing on chest exam	• COPD (p. 17) • Acute bronchospasms • Pulmonary embolism
	Abnormal EKG	• Ischemia • Arrhythmias • Heart failure

continued

Diagnostic Chart for Conditions of Aging *continued*

Clinical Manifestations	Concurrent Finding	Diagnosis Considerations
	Decreased hematocrit, pallor	• Anemia
	Elevated ESR or positive ANA	• System lupus erythematosis (SLE) other connective tissue disease • Rheumatologic disorder
	Elevated or low glucose	• Diabetes mellitus or insipidus • Hypoglycemia
	Elevated sugar	• Diabetes mellitus or insipidus
	Icterus, elevated LFTs	• Hepatitis • Cirrhosis
	Occult blood in stool	• Anemia
	Thyroid function test abnormality	• Hyper- or hypothyroidism
Gait abnormalities	Dementia and urinary incontinence	• Normal pressure hydrocephalus
	Malnutrition	• Vitamin B_{12} deficiency
	Neck pain and stiffness, numbness or tingling in arms	• Ankylosing spondylitis
	Pain, swelling, stiffness in joints	• Osteoarthritis (p. 77) • Rheumatoid arthritis
	Poor diet	• Nutrition deficiency
	Precipitating medications (e.g., phenthiazines, alphamethyldopa, many antipsychotics)	• Parkinson-like changes
	Progressive loss of strength and limb coordination, cramps	• Amyotrophic lateral scoliosis
	Progressive muscle wasting, weakness, loss of mobility	• Muscular dystrophy
	Symptoms appear and disappear	• Multiple sclerosis
	Abnormal "get up and go" test	• Gait or balance disturbance • Myopathy • Arthritis • Parkinson's disease (p. 91) • Postural hypotension • Poor conditioning

continued

Diagnostic Chart for Conditions of Aging *continued*

Clinical Manifestations	Concurrent Finding	Diagnosis Considerations
	Accompanied by other neurologic findings	• Organic brain lesion (e.g., subdural hematoma, brain tumor, normal pressure hydrocephalus, multi-infarct dementia)
	Degeneration of hip muscles	• Myositis • Polymyalgia rheumatica
	Diminished joint ROM	• Musculoskeletal disease
	Hand tremor, slowness and stiffness, loss of balance, autonomic dysfunction	• Parkinson's disease (p. 91)
	Hearing deficit, tinnitus	• Ear disorders (e.g., acoustic neuroma) • Meniere's disease
	Irregular steps, veering side to side	• Chronic alcoholism • Multiple sclerosis • Cerebral tumor • Vascular event
	Leg swings outward, localized loss of muscle strength	• Cerebrovascular accident
	Loss of sensation, muscle weakness	• Spinal cord trauma • Spinal tumor
	Papilledema	• Subdural hematoma or brain tumor
	Poor vision	• Environmental isolation
	Positive Romberg test (instability mostly with eyes closed)	• Sensory deficits • Poor proprioception
	Unsteadiness when sternum is pushed	• Parkinson's disease (p. 91) • Normal pressure hydrocephalus • Central nervous system disease • Osteoarthritis of lower back
	Unsteady when turning	• Parkinson's disease (p. 91) • Sensory defects • Cerebellar disease

continued

Diagnostic Chart for Conditions of Aging *continued*

Clinical Manifestations	Concurrent Finding	Diagnosis Considerations
		• Vision loss • Ataxia
	Leukocytosis	• Infection
Hypertension	Atonic bladder, tingling or numbness in lower extremities	• Diabetic autonomic neuropathy • Low spinal cord lesions
	Difficult to control with antihypertensive medications	• Renovascular hypertension (p. 61) • Hyperthyroidism
	Alternate between normal and high blood pressure	• Labile hypertension (p. 61)
	Blood pressure high in clinical setting but normal at home	• "White coat" hypertension (p. 61)
	Elevation of systolic pressure only	• Systolic hypertension (p. 61)
	Hyperlipidemia, type 2 diabetes mellitus	• Syndrome X
	Hypotensive symptoms before normalization of blood pressure	• Pseudohypertension (p. 61)
	Tremor, weight loss, increased appetite	• Hyperthyroidism
	Abnormal EKG	• Ischemia • Arrhythmias • CHF (p. 1) • Cardiac hypertrophy
	Increased red blood cell mass	• Polycythemia vera
	Positive captopril renal scan	• Renovascular hypertension
	Thyroid function test abnormality	• Hyper- or hypothyroidism
Inability to control urinary habits	Dementia, physical limitation	• Functional incontinence (p. 103)
	Desire to void occurs only when bladder is full	• Decreased bladder sensitivity
	Heavy caffeine, fluid intake	• Fluid excess

continued

Diagnostic Chart for Conditions of Aging *continued*

Clinical Manifestations	Concurrent Finding		Diagnosis Considerations
	Large volume urine loss with urgency		• Urge incontinence (p. 103)
	Mixed volume loss associated with nonbladder/nonurinary system disease		• Functional incontinence (p. 103)
	Muscle stiffness, fatigue or external dyspnea		• Dysmobility disorder
	Persistent urinary incontinence		• Stress incontinence (p. 103) • Urgency incontinence (p. 103) • Overflow incontinence (p. 103) • Functional incontinence (p. 103) • Mixed incontinence (p. 103)
	Reduced cognition		• Dementia (p. 29)
	Small volume urine loss	Associated with increased intra-abdominal pressure (sneeze, severe, standing)	• Stress incontinence (p. 103)
		With distended bladder	• Overflow incontinence (p. 103)
	Sudden need to urinate, frequent urination		• Irritable bladder (p. 103) • Urge incontinence (p. 103)
	Transient duration (less than 1 month)		• Delirium • Infection • Atrophic urethritis/vaginitis • Pharmaceuticals • Psychologic • Endocrine • Restricted mobility • Fecal impaction
	Triad of dementia and urinary incontinence and gait disorder		• Normal pressure hydrocephalus
	Atrophic urethritis, atrophic vaginitis, gradual onset of symptoms		• Estrogen withdrawal
	Decrease flexion and extension strength of ankle, knee and hip, decreased rectal sphincter tone		• S2, S3, S4 neuropathy or cord lesion

continued

Diagnostic Chart for Conditions of Aging *continued*

Clinical Manifestations	Concurrent Finding	Diagnosis Considerations
	Distended jugular veins, dependent edema, pulmonary rales, enlarged heart, an S3 gallop	• CHF (p. 1)
	Enlarged bladder	• Overflow incontinence (p. 103)
	Pelvic abnormality on exam	• Dry vaginal mucosa • Pelvic or rectal masses • Uterine prolapse • Cystocele
	Blood in urine	• Tumor • Infection • Stone disease
	Elevated or low glucose	• Diabetes mellitus or insipidus • Hypoglycemia
	Post-void residual is elevated (greater than 200 mL)	• Prostate enlargement • Bladder muscle dysfunction • Bladder tumor
	Protein in urine	• Renal disease • Diabetes mellitus
	White blood cell in urine with bacteria	• Urinary tract infection
Insomnia	Daytime sleeping	• Change in sleep habits
	Difficulty falling asleep and/or anxious feeling	• Anxiety disorder • Thyroid disease • Inactivity during day • Transient situational insomnia • Exercise/fluid intake close to bedtime • Chronic pain (e.g., HA, GI, arthritis) • Depression (p. 43)
	Early morning wakening, depressed mood, anhedonia, diminished energy/concentration/appetite	• Major depression • Thyroid disease
	Fatigue, decreased appetite, apathy	• Depression (p. 43)
	Frequent awakening	• Sleep apnea

continued

Diagnostic Chart for Conditions of Aging *continued*

Clinical Manifestations	Concurrent Finding	Diagnosis Considerations
	Loud snoring	• Hypothyroidism • Sleep apnea • Obesity/Pickwickian syndrome
	New nightmares	• Emotional distress • Hypoglycemia • Anoxia • Medication side effect
	Nocturia	• BPH or other urethral obstruction • Diabetes mellitus or insipidus • CHF (p. 1) • Renal insufficiency • Cirrhosis with ascites
	Nocturnal episodes of shortness of breath	• Paroxysmal nocturnal dyspnea
	Palpitations	• Hyperthyroidism • Mitral valve prolapse • Anxiety disorder • Tachyarrhythmias
	Poor sleep quality	• Caffeine use • Medications, such as psychotropics, beta blockers, sympathomimetics, diuretics, hypnotics • Painful, uncomfortable conditions and changes in sleep habits of older adults, • Anxiety • Depression (p. 43)
	"Restless" or twitching legs	• Nocturnal myoclonus • Restless leg syndrome
	Somatic complaints	• Anxiety disorder • Organic disease • Somatoform disorder
	Substance or chronic medication use	• Alcohol/drug related insomnia • Tolerance to sleep medications

continued

Diagnostic Chart for Conditions of Aging *continued*

Clinical Manifestations	Concurrent Finding	Diagnosis Considerations
	Arousal during REM	• Nightmares • Night terrors
Joint pain/stiffness	Fatigue and malaise	• Rheumatoid arthritis • Polymyalgia rheumatica • Joint infection
	Involvement of proximal interphalangeal joints	• Osteoarthritis (p. 77)
	Morning stiffness, usually less than 30 minutes duration	• Osteoarthritis (p. 77)
	Anemia	• Rheumatoid arthritis • Polymyalgia rheumatica
	Fever	• Gout • Hepatitis • Infectious arthritis • Viral syndrome • Lyme disease • Osteomyelitis • Rheumatoid arthritis • Sarcoidosis • Syphilis • SLE • Tendinitis
	Joint erythema and warmth	• Rheumatoid arthritis • Gout • Pseudogout • Joint infection
	Joint motion leads to sensations or sound of popping or grinding	• Osteoarthritis (p. 77)
	Minimal signs of acute inflammation	• Osteoarthritis (p. 77)
	Muscle tenderness	• Polymyalgia rheumatica
	Nonjoint findings	• Polymyalgia rheumatica • Joint infection • Rheumatoid arthritis

continued

Diagnostic Chart for Conditions of Aging *continued*

Clinical Manifestations	Concurrent Finding	Diagnosis Considerations
		• Psoriasis • Collagen disease
	Symmetrical joint involvement	• Rheumatoid arthritis • Polymyalgia rheumatica
	Wrist involvement	• Rheumatoid arthritis
	Elevated sugar	• Diabetes mellitus or insipidus
	Elevated white blood cell, ESR	• Rheumatoid arthritis • Polymyalgia rheumatica • Joint infection
Memory loss/forgetfulness	Acute onset, days to weeks	• Drug-induced thyroid disease • Subdural etiology • Metabolic disorder
	Choreiform movements	• Huntington's disease
	Decreased appetite, swollen abdomen and/or legs, itching	• Cirrhosis
	Drug or toxin exposure, dietary deficiency	• Alcohol dementia • Narcotic/toxin poisoning • Thiamin deficiency • Vitamin B_{12} deficiency
	Fatigue, weight gain	• Hypothyroidism
	Hallucinations	• Substance abuse • Lewy body variant dementia • Psychosis
	Headache, vomiting	• Brain tumor • Increased intracranial pressure
	Hearing loss	• Social isolation
	Low self-esteem, feeling blue	• Wilson's disease
	Nonprogressive, little effect on functional ability	• Age-associated memory impairment (p. 30)
	Recent drug withdrawal (e.g., benzodiazepines, alcohol)	• Drug withdrawal-induced brain dysfunction

continued

Diagnostic Chart for Conditions of Aging *continued*

Clinical Manifestations	Concurrent Finding	Diagnosis Considerations
	Recent history of head trauma	• Subdural hematoma
	Slowly progressive symptoms over more than 6 months	• Alzheimer's disease (p. 29)
	Slurred speech, weakness of extremities, incontinence	• Multiple sclerosis
	Stepwise deterioration with plateaus	• Multi-infarct dementia (p. 29)
	Sudden onset	• Intracranial pathology • Metabolic abnormalities • Substance abuse • Medication-induced • Thyroid disease • Bereavement
	Sudden paralysis, loss of sensation, speech abnormalities	• Cerebrovascular accident
	Use of benzodiazepines, hypnotic or other psychotropics, use of potentially offending medications (e.g., anticholinergics, sedatives, hypnotics)	• Medication-induced forgetfulness
	Younger age, rapidly progressive, associated neurologic abnormalities	• Creutzfeldt-Jakob disease
	Accompanied by other focal neurologic findings	• Organic brain lesion (e.g., subdural hematoma, brain tumor, normal pressure hydrocephalus, multi-infarct dementia)
	Evidence of infection	• HIV • Syphilis • Granulomatous disease • Other viral/fungal/protozoan disease • Meningitis • Encephalitis • Sepsis
	Evidence of vascular disease	• Multi-infarct dementia (p. 29) • Vasculitis • Subcortical dementia (p. 29)

continued

Diagnostic Chart for Conditions of Aging *continued*

Clinical Manifestations	Concurrent Finding	Diagnosis Considerations
	Hearing deficit, tinnitus	• Ear disorders
	Inadequate fluid intake	• Dehydration
	Increased respiratory rate	• CHF (p. 1) • Pneumonia • Early sepsis
	Motor and/or sensory function deficits	• Neurologic system disease
	Movement disorder/gait disturbance	• Parkinson's disease (p. 91) • Huntington's disease • Lewy body variant dementia • Creutzfeldt-Jakob disease (syndrome) • Hydrocephalus • Brain tumor • Alzheimer's disease (p. 29)
	Normal exam and labs	• Major depression (p. 43) • Anxiety disorder • Alzheimer's disease (p. 29)
	Papilledema	• Subdural hematoma or brain tumor
	Progressive decrease in cognitive skills	• Alzheimer's disease (p. 29) • Multi-infarct dementia (p. 29) • Other progressive dementing processes (p. 29)
	Triad of dementia, gait disturbance and urinary incontinence	• Normal pressure hydrocephalus
	Abnormal EKG	• Ischemia • Arrhythmias • CHF (p. 1)
	Anemia, macrocytosis and/or hyper-segmented polymorphonucleocytes	• B_{12} deficiency
	Elevated or low glucose	• Diabetes mellitus or insipidus • Hypoglycemia
	Hypocalcemia	• Hyperparathyroidism • Multiple myeloma • Sarcoidosis

continued

Diagnostic Chart for Conditions of Aging *continued*

Clinical Manifestations	Concurrent Finding	Diagnosis Considerations
	Hypoxia	• COPD (p. 17) • CHF (p. 1) • Pneumonia • Pulmonary embolism
	Increased serum iron	• Hemochromatosis
	Leukocytosis	• Infection
	Thyroid function test abnormality	• Hyper- or hypothyroidism
Nausea and vomiting	Abdominal pain	• Gastrointestinal obstruction • Gastroenteritis • Hepatitis • Pancreatitis • Cholecystitis/cholelithiasis • Parasites • Diverticular disorders • Adrenal insufficiency • Disseminated intravascular coagulation • Endometriosis • Irritable bowel syndrome • Lactose intolerance • Peritonitis • Testicular torsion • Food poisoning • Leukemia
	Chest pain	• Myocardial infarction • Esophageal rupture • Strangulated diaphragmatic hernia • Coronary artery disease
	Diarrhea, acute onset	• Gastroenteritis
	Early-morning vomiting	• Alcohol ingestion • Uremia • Esophageal obstruction • Achalasia
	Headache	• Brain tumor or abscess • Trauma • Glaucoma

continued

Diagnostic Chart for Conditions of Aging *continued*

Clinical Manifestations	Concurrent Finding	Diagnosis Considerations
		• Hydrocephalus • Migraine • Meningitis • Food poisoning • Leukemia
	Hematemesis	• Gastritis • Esophageal varices • Gastric ulcer
	Medications (e.g., digitalis, theo-phylline, quinidine, antibiotics, NSAIDs)	• Medication effects
	Melancholia	• Depression (p. 43)
	Occurs when recumbent	• Posterior fossa lesion
	Preceded by cough	• Asthma
	Projectile vomiting, no nausea	• Increased intracranial pressure
	Shortness of breath, fatigue, ankle swelling	• CHF (p. 1)
	Vertigo and/or tinnitus	• Middle ear disorder • Meniere's disease • Labyrinthine disorder • Benign paroxysmal vertigo
	Distended abdomen	• Paralytic ileus • Mechanical bowel obstruction
	Fever, acute onset	• Infection
	Jaundice or hepatomegaly	• Hepatitis • Cirrhosis • Liver tumors
	Tachypnea	• Diabetic lactoacidosis
	Weight loss, no other signs or symptoms	• Anorexia nervosa
	Low red blood cell mass	• Anemia
Pedal edema, bilateral	Dyspnea on exertion	• Pericarditis

continued

Diagnostic Chart for Conditions of Aging *continued*

Clinical Manifestations	Concurrent Finding	Diagnosis Considerations
		• Valvular heart disease • CHF (p. 1) • Amyloidosis • COPD (p. 17)
	Impaired mobility	• Dependent position
	Poor diet	• Hypoproteinemia
	Use of estrogens, NSAIDs, psycho-tropic drugs, vasodilators, corticosteroids, methyldopa, hydralazine	• Fluid-retaining medications
	Generalized edema	• Nephrotic syndrome • Renal failure
	No evidence of organic disease	• Salt-retaining drugs • Dependent positioning • Constricting clothes
	Spider angiomas, hepatomegaly	• Cirrhosis
Shortness of breath	Acute onset	• Viral or bacterial infections, cardiac disease
	Chest pain	• Atelectasis • Cardiomyopathy • COPD (p. 17) • Pneumonia • Lung cancer • Myocardial infarction • Pericarditis • Pleuritis • Pneumothorax • Pulmonary embolism • Tuberculosis
	Dyspnea	• COPD (p. 17) • CHF (p. 1) • Pulmonary hypertension (p. 61) • Sarcoidosis • Pulmonary embolism

continued

Diagnostic Chart for Conditions of Aging *continued*

Clinical Manifestations	Concurrent Finding		Diagnosis Considerations
	History of cigarette smoking		• COPD (p. 17) • Lung cancer
	Lethargy, restlessness and/or mental status changes		• CHF (p. 1) • Pulmonary embolism • Acute myocardial infarct • Pneumonia
	Without clear cardiopulmonary disease		• Amyloidosis • Diphtheria • Leukemia • Anemia • Liver tumors • Myasthenia gravis • Nephrotic syndrome • Obesity • Renal failure
	Chronic limitation to expiratory airflow	With chronic productive cough	• Chronic bronchitis (p. 17)
		With wheezing and minimal cough and sputum production	• Emphysema (p. 17)
	Decreased breath sounds, hyperresonance of the chest		• COPD (p. 17)
	Distended jugular veins, dependent edema, pulmonary rales, pedal edema		• CHF (p. 1)
	Enlarged heart, an S3 gallop		• CHF (p. 1)
	Increased respiratory rate		• CHF (p. 1) • Pneumonia • Early sepsis • Pulmonary embolism • Pneumothorax
	Resting tachycardia		• CHF (p. 1) • Arrhythmia

continued

Diagnostic Chart for Conditions of Aging *continued*

Clinical Manifestations	Concurrent Finding	Diagnosis Considerations
		• Anemia • Pulmonary embolism • Pneumonia
	Wheezing on chest exam	• COPD (p. 17) • Acute bronchospasms
	Abnormal EKG	• Ischemia • Arrhythmias • CHF (p. 1) • Myocarditis • Endocarditis • Pericardial effusion
	Occult blood in stool	• Anemia
	Pedal edema	• CHF (p. 1) • Ischemic heart disease
Terminal illness	Abdominal pain, bloating, nausea, urinary incontinence	• Constipation
	Dyspnea	• Anxiety • Pain • CHF (p. 1) • COPD (p. 17) • Pneumonia • Hypoxia • Other noncardiopulmonary disease
	Fear, anger, agitation	• Anxiety • Delirium • Dementia (p. 29)
	Nausea	• Medications • Constipation • Gastric irritation • Underlying disease process
	Pain	• Anxiety • Depression (p. 43) • Fear • Fatigue

continued

Diagnostic Chart for Conditions of Aging *continued*

Clinical Manifestations	Concurrent Finding	Diagnosis Considerations
		• Loneliness • Inflammation • Immobilization
	Poor diet	• Nutrition deficiency
	Urinary retention/incontinence	• Enlarged prostate • Impacted stool • Bladder atony • Intrinsic bladder disease • Neurogenic bladder • Urinary tract infection
	Vomiting	• Medications • GI obstruction • Brain metastasis • Metabolic abnormalities
	Anorexia and poor nutrition	• Lack of interest in eating • Lack of appetite • Loss of control • Medication reactions • Poor fitting dentures • Esophageal infections or dysmobility • Gastric irritation • Tumor-related problems
Tremor	Antecedent dementia	• Alzheimer's disease (p. 29)
	Appear then disappear, weakness in extremities	• Multiple sclerosis
	Does not fit any regular pattern	• Drug abuse • Somatization disorder
	Headaches, nausea and vomiting	• Brain tumors
	Hunger, anxiety, trembling, perspiration	• Hypoglycemia
	Occurs with intentional movement	• Cerebellar disease • Wilson's disease • Multiple sclerosis
	Precipitating medications	• Parkinson-like changes

continued

Diagnostic Chart for Conditions of Aging *continued*

Clinical Manifestations	Concurrent Finding	Diagnosis Considerations
	(e.g., phenthiazines, alphamethyldopa, many antipsychotics)	
	Sudden onset of fear and panic, palpitations	• Anxiety disorder
	Worsened by coffee, drugs, nicotine, fatigue	• Enhanced physiologic tremor • Hyperthyroidism • Hypoglycemia • Alcohol or drug withdrawal
	Hand tremor, slowness and stiffness, loss of balance, autonomic dysfunction	• Parkinson's disease (p. 91)
	Low-amplitude, high-frequency tremor aggravated by specific factors (e.g., stress, caffeine, fatigue)	• Psychologic tremor
	Low-frequency tremor increasing with age, worsening with movement	• Essential tremor
	Masked facies	• Parkinson's disease (p. 91)
	Movement disorders looking like tremors	• Asterixis • Myoclonus • Fasciculations
	Proximal tremor with liver disease	• Wilson's disease
	Weight loss, increased appetite	• Hyperthyroidism
	Thyroid function test elevated or low	• Hyper- or hypothyroidism
Weight Loss	Abdominal pain	• Adrenal insufficiency • Intestinal parasite • Colitis • Colon cancer • Pancreatic cancer • Crohn's disease • Leukemia • Pancreatitis • Peptic ulcer • Stomach cancer • Uterine cancer

continued

Diagnostic Chart for Conditions of Aging *continued*

Clinical Manifestations	Concurrent Finding	Diagnosis Considerations
	Anorexia	• Poor dentures • Dementia (p. 29) • Depression (p. 43) • Anxiety • GI disorders • Aging process • Other organic disorders
	Decreased appetite, nausea, swollen legs, confusion	• Cirrhosis
	Dysphagia, regurgitation of food	• Esophageal cancer • Esophageal obstruction
	Environmental factors	• Recent relocation • Bereavement • Inadequate socialization
	Fatigue, thirst, frequent urination, good appetite	• Diabetes mellitus
	Insomnia, fatigue, sleep disorder	• Depression (p. 43)
	Normal appetite	• Diabetes mellitus • AIDS • Hyperthyroidism • Decreased intestinal absorption • Overactivity
	Shortness of breath	• CHF (p. 1) • Sarcoidosis • Pneumonia • Tuberculosis • COPD (p. 17)
	Use of offending medicines, drowsiness, dry mouth, nausea	• Medication effects
	Diffuse lymphadenopathy	• Lymphoma
	Fever	• Infection
	Tingling, numbness, muscle weakness	• Peripheral neuropathy
	Anemia	• Folic acid deficiency • Pernicious anemia
	Increased red blood cell mass	• Polycythemia vera

INTRODUCTION

....

CARING FOR OUR ELDERS

As we approach the next century, the largest-growing segment of our population is comprised of those age 85 or older. We as a society face a future with more seniors in our country than at any time in our history. The social, political, and financial world that has defined us will change. The health needs of this group will unceasingly demand more attention. The practice of the current and near-future family physicians will increasingly focus on providing health care for this age group.

The focus of geriatric medicine is different from the focus of internal medicine. Medical illnesses and disease diagnosis and management take a place on the back burner. The patients' functional status must be the major concern. It matters less the exact cause of elderly patients' heart failure or renal failure; it is more important to know if they can obtain their own food, prepare themselves meals, or get to the bathroom or if they have any tendencies to fall. The patients' cholesterol level or sedimentation rate are less valuable indicators of morbidity or mortality than their point score on a mental-status testing. Geriatric functional assessment is the cornerstone of good health care for seniors. Physical assessment must include an evaluation of a patient's activities of daily living (ADLs) and instrumental activities of daily living (IADLs). Every elderly patient should be assessed for urinary incontinence, falls, and mental status. This book is focused on the top 10 diagnoses that present to a family physician's office, and each of these issues are addressed as they relate to these presentations.

Overall, medication use in the elderly is plagued with a myriad of complications and side effects. All medications should be started at as low a dose as possible and titrated slowly to their desired effect. It is frequently the case that the best drug for the job is no drug at all. Discontinuing medications may produce significant improvements in a patient's physical and mental status. I was told by my mentor, Alex Comfort, M.D., a renowned British geriatrician, that I could ensure my success as a physician for the elderly over my career by stopping more medicines than I started. "Start low and go slow" and "Stop more medicines than you start" should be on the front of your sample cabinets and prescription pads.

Lastly, let me suggest that care of the elderly involves an aggressive, not passive, approach to end-of-life care. The chapter in this text that means the most to me is the chapter on terminal-illness care. I find that all too often the issues concerning end-of-life care are not addressed until the end of life is rapidly approaching. Humans age slowly, and we have thoughts of our death as we pass landmarks such as thirtieth, fortieth, or fiftieth birthdays or sentinel events such as a child's graduation or marriage. We look to the future and hope to make it to the next decade or the next events. Physicians, however, have a tendency not to discuss end-of-life issues with patients until they become really sick. We should make these discussions a part of routine care for elders and, for that matter, for all patients. Everyone should have an advanced directive. Everyone should have a plan for their care should they become incapacitated and have to live the remainder of their lives without cognitive function and with artificial feedings. Family physicians should be at the center of the issues involving end-of-life care.

THE AAFP QUICK REFERENCE GUIDE

When I entered the study of geriatrics 13 years ago, I was confronted by a group of academicians who wanted to train only those physicians who would be university-based research faculty. In fact, the only "fellowships in geriatrics" available until 1996 were 2 years in length with a full year of required research. The education of the practicing family physician was viewed by these academic subspecialists as unnecessary, since clearly all patients would be referred into the university centers or to multidisciplinary teams headed by geriatric specialists. These were ideas that would clearly fail.

I found solace in a few internists and family physicians who understood the role of the practicing family physician in the health care of the elderly. The time had come to disseminate the new information generated about the care of the elderly to family physicians. The American Academy of Family Physicians, with the leadership of their Director of the Division of Education at the time, Jane Murray, M.D., took on the task of providing nationwide education for family physicians on caring for our elders. Thus was born an annual AAFP CME entitled "Geriatric Review Course for Family Physicians." This manual is an extension of these beginnings. These chapters were constructed for practicing family physicians as they care for elderly patients in their offices. The content was not meant to be exhaustive nor does it contain all the background research in the field of geriatrics. It is not meant to replace any authoritative textbook in geriatrics. It is meant to provide concise advice to aid busy family physicians in their daily work.

Over the last 10 years I have taught family physicians across the United States about the care of the elderly. I have always focused on trying to make the complex issues usable for the office practice of family medicine. Attendees at these meetings would frequently ask for a textbook that would help them in their practice, and I have referred them to references that I use as a teacher. However, I know that for most of their needs these texts have far too much material that will only hinder in their search for quick answers. Such utility is the goal of this new AAFP Quick Reference Guide.

The topics in this book are the most common diagnoses/complaints of the elderly in a family practice. By design, there are no chapters on hospital care or nursing-home care. Each chapter is organized as the patient would be evaluated by his or her doctor, starting with chief complaint, data collection through history, physical and diagnostic tests, formulating a differential diagnosis, treatment, follow-up, and patient education.

I hope that you find this format useful and that it aids you in making the care of the elderly a pleasure for you. Our patients deserve our finest efforts.

Lanyard K. Dial, MD

Congestive Heart Failure

Congestive heart failure (CHF), defined as reduced cardiac function causing inadequate circulation of blood to meet the metabolic needs of the body, has been increasing in frequency among elderly adults. It is the most frequent discharge diagnosis of hospitalized Medicare beneficiaries. Reduced cardiac function caused by ventricular dysfunction can be either systolic failure (inadequate cardiac output from lack of systolic contractile forces) or isolated diastolic failure (inadequate cardiac output from the insufficient filling of the ventricle during diastole). The concept of isolated diastolic dysfunction is almost totally unique to CHF in the elderly, and its understanding is essential to patient management. Diastolic dysfunction results from impaired left ventricular relaxation and reduced compliance, whereas systolic dysfunction is a decrease in contractile ability of the left ventricle causing a decreased ejection fraction.

Although the causes of CHF are similar among all age groups, almost 80% of cases of CHF in elderly patients are the result of hypertension or coronary artery disease. The increasing prevalence of long-standing hypertension and coronary artery disease in the aging population, as well as age-related changes in cardiac function, is responsible for the increasing frequency of this cardiac disorder.

CHIEF COMPLAINT

The older adult with CHF, who is probably more sedentary than a younger person, will not notice symptoms early in the progression of cardiac dysfunction. The clinical presentation of CHF in the elderly is frequently different from the classic symptoms (Table 1.1). Exertional dyspnea is often masked by the sedentary lifestyle of the elderly and is often explained away by the patient as a consequence of aging instead of as a disease. In fact, dyspnea in the elderly is more commonly related to chronic obstructive pulmonary disease (COPD) than to CHF, and pedal edema is most often a manifestation of venous insufficiency rather than CHF.

Other common presenting complaints in the elderly person with CHF are anorexia, insomnia, nocturnal cough, and nocturia. Patients with comorbid conditions that put more pressure on cardiac function, including hypertension, fluid retention from renal disease or medications, anemia, thyroid disease, and febrile illnesses causing increased cardiac output, will present with symptoms at earlier stages of myocardial dysfunction.

HISTORY

The patient's history will provide insight into the underlying etiology and the precipitating causes of CHF, as well as the patient's current level of functioning (Table 1.2).

A detailed past medical history is important, including previous cardiac diseases, alcohol use, and thyroid or malignant disorders, and can help determine the underlying cause. Comorbid illnesses and conditions should be identified. Historical facts can also lead to the precipitating factor for the acute crisis. The following can be key factors in CHF: taking medications that have a negative effect on cardiac output (calcium channel blockers, β-blockers, and some antiarrhythmics); taking medications that increase intravascular volume (nonsteroidal, anti-inflammatory agents [NSAIDs] or hormonal agents); not taking medications that are prescribed to be beneficial (diuretics, angiotensin-converting enzyme [ACE] inhibitors, nitrates); or not taking prescribed medications correctly. The classic geriatric case is the patient placed on a new ophthalmologic drop for glaucoma (a β-blocker) that precipitates an episode of heart failure. New ischemia should always be considered (Tables 1.3 and 1.4).

TABLE 1.1. Clinical Complaints with CHF

Classic Presentation	Presentation in the Elderly
Dyspnea	Lethargy
Pedal edema	Restlessness
	Mental status changes

TABLE 1.2. Questions about Current Illness

Ankle swelling
Dyspnea, at rest, on exertion
Exercise intolerance
Fatigue
Lethargy
Medication use
Mental status changes
Orthopnea
Restlessness

TABLE 1.3. **Potential Etiologies of Congestive Heart Failure**

Congenital cardiomyopathy
Diabetes
Hypertensive cardiomyopathy
Infectious cardiomyopathy
Ischemic cardiomyopathy
Metabolic cardiomyopathy (thyroid disorders, amyloid infiltration, sarcoidosis)
Myocardial neoplasm (atrial myxoma)
Pericardial restriction
Toxic cardiomyopathy (alcohol, anthracyclines)
Valvular heart disease

TABLE 1.4. **Precipitating Causes of Congestive Heart Failure**

Acute or chronic blood loss
Alterations in thyroid, renal disease
Arrhythmias
Exacerbation or development of underlying medical illness
Excessive salt and fluid intake
Infections
Medications (poor compliance, negative inotropic agents, preload reduction in diastolic failure)
New ischemia or infarction

PHYSICAL EXAMINATION

The physical examination is important in patients in whom CHF is suspected, as well as in patients with CHF, to determine the severity of the illness. The physical exam may also indicate the underlying cause of the CHF and the precipitating factors. Physical findings will differ in patients with underlying systolic versus isolated diastolic heart failure. A complete physical examination is also essential for determining comorbid conditions and complications secondary to heart failure.

Cardiac Examination

- Systolic CHF: Enlarged cardiac borders, a displaced point of maximal impulse, an S3 gallop, and a resting tachycardia.
- Diastolic CHF: Normal cardiac borders, a sustained point of maximal impulse, and occasionally an S4 heart sound.
- Exercise patient mildly in office, watching for DOE and raised pulse rate.

Noncardiac Exam

- Systolic CHF: Patients will have distension of the jugular veins, a diminished carotid upstroke, poor peripheral perfusion, dependent edema, and pulmonary rales.
- Diastolic dysfunction: Patients will likely be hypertensive, will show evidence of arterial insufficiency, and will not have jugular distension.

DIAGNOSTIC TEST DATA

Diagnostic tests are essential for diagnosis and management of patients with CHF. Patients with symptoms that are highly suggestive of heart failure should have echocardiography to measure left ventricular ejection fraction (EF) even if the physical signs of heart failure are absent. The Agency for Health Care Policy and Research (AHCPR) has released recommendations on management of heart failure; Table 1.5 lists the recommended tests for initial evaluation.

- Resting Electrocardiogram. The electrocardiogram (ECG) is fundamental as it gives important information about cardiac rate, rhythm, axis, hypertrophy, and signs of disease such as ischemia, infarction, and pericardial fluid and inflammation. Every patient with CHF should have a resting ECG on an annual basis, as well as with the occurrence of any exacerbation.
- Echocardiography. These studies are far more accurate than the physical exam or any other laboratory test in determining cardiac chamber size, valvular diseases, and even cardiac muscular function. Every patient with CHF should have one of these studies early after initial diagnosis and periodically throughout management. Echocardiography is the most definitive way to differentiate systolic from diastolic CHF. These tests help to determine the severity of systolic CHF by providing quantitative measurements of the ejection fraction, as well as information about ventricular wall motion. Echocardiography is readily available, and able to detect pericardial effusion and ventricular thrombus, but is sometimes technically inadequate and difficult to perform in patients with lung disease.
- Blood Tests. In the initial evaluation of a patient with CHF, blood testing should include a complete blood count (CBC), a chemistry panel to detect electrolytes and renal and hepatic function, and screening thyroid studies. Other tests should be done if indicated by additional findings in the database. Because most patients with CHF receive a diuretic, periodic reevaluation of serum electrolytes and renal function is critical. Monitoring drug levels such as in patients receiving digoxin is also important.
- Other tests. An initial, plain-film, chest radiograph can be helpful in looking

TABLE 1.5. **AHCPR Recommended Tests for Patients with Signs or Symptoms of Heart Failure**

Test Recommendation	Finding	Suspected Diagnosis
Electrocardiogram	Acute ST-T wave changes	Myocardial ischemia
	Atrial fibrillation, other tachyarrhythmias	Thyroid disease or heart failure due to rapid ventricular rate
	Bradyarrhythmias	Heart failure due to low heart rate
	Previous MI (e.g., Q waves)	Heart failure due to reduced left-ventricular performance
	Low voltage	Pericardial effusion
	Left-ventricular hypertrophy	Diastolic dysfunction
Complete blood count	Anemia	Heart failure due to or aggravated by decreased oxygen-carrying capacity
Urinalysis	Proteinuria	Nephrotic syndrome
	Red blood cells or cellular casts	Glomerulonephritis
Serum creatinine	Elevated	Volume overload due to renal failure
Serum albumin	Decreased	Increased extravascular volume due to hypoalbuminemia
T4 and TSH (obtain only if atrial fibrillation, evidence of thyroid disease, or patient age > 65)	Abnormal T4 or TSH	Heart failure due to or aggravated by hypo/hyperthyroidism

Reprinted from Konstam M, Dracup K, Baker D, et al. Heart failure: management of patients with left-ventricular systolic dysfunction. Quick reference guide for clinicians no. 11. AHCPR publication no. 94–0613. Rockville, MD: Agency for Health Care Policy and Research, Public Health Service, U.S. Dept. of Health and Human Services, 1994.
MI, myocardial infarction; *TSH*, thyroid stimulating hormone.

at the cardiac silhouette and for pulmonary congestion. Chest radiographs may be obtained regularly and with the occurrence of exacerbations.

• Other cardiac testing. Tests such as Holter monitoring, radionuclide scans, or exercise tests have no direct role in the routine management of patients with CHF. These tests are reserved for specific indications such as undiagnosed rate/rhythm disturbances and for assessment of ischemic episodes. If angina or extensive ischemia is noted on these noninvasive tests, coronary angiography is useful in patients who are candidates for revascularization procedures.

DIFFERENTIAL DIAGNOSIS

CHF is a syndrome of clinical features that can be caused by a variety of underlying illnesses and made manifest by a variety of precipitating events. The diagnosis of CHF demands further investigation into the underlying etiology and the precipitating factors. The diagnosis also includes distinguishing systolic failure (inadequate cardiac output from lack of systolic contractile forces) from diastolic failure (inadequate cardiac output from insufficient filling of the ventricle during diastole) (Table 1.6).

WHEN TO REFER

The diagnosis and treatment of patients with CHF generally does not require referral or consultation. Consultation with a cardiologist or an internist may be helpful if the patient does not respond to the usual therapy or if the patient has a complex interaction of a number of diseases or medications.

MANAGEMENT

Management is dictated by the principles listed in Table 1.7. Figure 1.1 is an algorithm of management.

General Measures

The following measures should be taken in the treatment of CHF:

• Fluid intake should be kept to 1500 to 2000 mL per day; although fluid restriction is generally not advisable unless the patient develops hyponatremia.

TABLE 1.6. Systolic Versus Diastolic CHF

	Systolic CHF	Diastolic CHF
Pathophysiology	Dilated ventricle that cannot adequately pump blood forward to meet circulatory demand; inadequate cardiac pump	Hypertrophied ventricle that cannot adequately fill with blood so that its forward pump cannot meet circulatory demand; inadequate cardiac filling
Cardiac history	Previous myocardial infarctions (MIs)— especially anterior wall damage	Hypertension, coronary disease without MI
Echocardiogram	Dilated ventricular chambers, thin ventricular walls, poor ejection fraction (<40%)	Hypertrophied ventricular walls, small chamber size, normal ejection fraction (>40%)
Physical exam	Cardiomegaly, S3 gallop, tachycardia, raised jugular venous pressure	Small heart, S4 gallop

TABLE 1.7. Mechanisms for Improving CHF

SYSTOLIC CHF
Increase myocardial contractility (digoxin).
Reduce ventricular preload and pulmonary congestion (low sodium diet: <2 g, diuretics, nitrates).
Reduce afterload (ACE inhibitors, nitrates, and hydralazine).
Maintain sinus rhythm (digoxin, β-blockers[a]).
Reduce myocardial ischemia (nitrates, β-blockers[a]).

DIASTOLIC CHF
Improve left ventricular relaxation and reduce left ventricular mass.
ACE inhibitors, β-blockers, calcium channel blockers.
Reduce pulmonary congestion (low sodium diet, diuretics, nitrates).
Decrease elevated systolic blood pressure (diuretics, ACE inhibitors, β-blockers, calcium channel blockers).
Maintain sinus rhythm (digoxin).
Reduce myocardial ischemia (nitrates, β-blockers).
Slow ventricular rate (β-blockers, calcium channel blockers).

[a]Newer studies show potential benefits of β-blocker use in some patients with systolic heart failure.

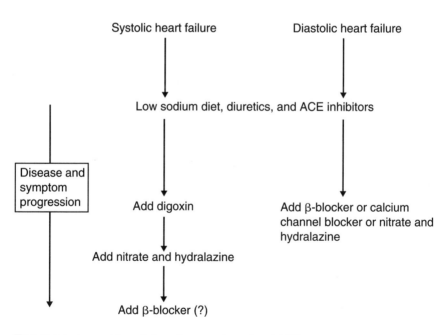

FIGURE 1.1. Heart failure therapy algorithm. (*ACE*, angiotensin-converting enzyme.)

- Alcohol use should be discouraged. Patients who drink alcohol should have no more than one drink per day.
- Regular physical activity should be encouraged as it will preserve functional abilities and improve the patient's quality of life. Even short periods of bed rest should be discouraged as they result in decreased exercise tolerance.
- Exacerbating medications should be watched carefully, especially those such as NSAIDs, which could worsen renal function.
- Sodium intake should be reduced to less than 3 to 4 g of sodium chloride per day. Elderly patients have decreased salt sensitivity and typically will utilize more salt to ensure adequate taste. Patients can be advised to use other spices and herbs to improve the taste of foods and thereby aid their compliance with sodium restriction.

Medications

Diuretics

Diuretics should be thought of as first-line agents in the treatment of patients with either systolic or diastolic CHF (Table 1.8). They are especially useful in patients with clear evidence of volume overload. Diuretics decrease total body fluid, reduce ventricular preload, and thereby reduce pulmonary congestion and edema. Reducing preload is essential in patients with poor left ventricular function. Judicious diuretic use can also benefit older adults with diastolic dysfunction and a normal left ventricular ejection fraction. However, excessive diuresis in these patients will exacerbate CHF.

Many patients can achieve adequate therapy with a mild thiazide-type diuretic, others will need a loop diuretic such as furosemide (Lasix), and some will require the addition of metolazone (Mykrox, Zaroxolyn) to their regimens. Metolazone plus a loop diuretic produces a significant diuresis in even the most severe cases. However, this combination is also notorious for precipitating dehydration and severe hyponatremia if not watched carefully.

TABLE 1.8. Diuretics in the Treatment of Congestive Heart Failure

Diuretic	Dosage
Hydrochlorothiazide (Esidrix)	25 to 50 mg daily
Chlorthalidone (Hygroton)	25 to 50 mg daily
Furosemide (Lasix)	10 to 80 mg daily
Spironolactone (Aldactone)	25 to 200 mg daily
Triamterene (Dyrenium)	50 to 200 mg daily
Amiloride (Midamor)	5 to 20 mg daily
Metolazone (Diulo)	2.5 to 10 mg daily

TABLE 1.9.   ACE Inhibitor Use in Patients with Congestive Heart Failure

ACE Inhibitor	Initial Dosing	Target Dosing	Maximal Dosing
Captopril (Capoten)	6.25 mg three times daily	50 mg three times daily	100 mg three times daily
Enalapril (Vasotec)	2.5 mg two times daily	10 mg two times daily	20 mg two times daily
Benazepril (Lotensin)	5 mg one time daily	20 mg one time daily	40 mg one time daily
Lisinopril (Zestril)	2.5–5 mg one time daily	20 mg one time daily	40 mg one time daily
Quinapril (Accupril)	5 mg one time daily	20 mg two times daily	20 mg two times daily
Fosinopril (Monopril)	10 mg one time daily	20 mg one time daily	40 mg one time daily
Ramipril (Altace)	2.5 mg one time daily	10 mg one time daily (5 mg two times daily)	20 mg two times daily

Side Effects.   Older adults have a narrow, therapeutic window for diuretics. Even with small doses, excessive diuresis can result in dehydration, hypotension, and azotemia problems that may be exacerbated by the addition of ACE inhibitors. Electrolyte disturbances from diuretics are also more common in the elderly. Both sodium and potassium balances can be disturbed by diuretics. Diuretic choices will depend on the severity of the patient's CHF and on the patient's renal function.

ACE Inhibitors

ACE inhibitors should be standard therapy in all patients with CHF because of their proven ability to improve survival in such patients. They are also very effective in reducing symptoms, increasing exercise tolerance, and improving functional status and quality of life. Unless there is a clear contraindication (such as evidence of renal toxicity, hyperkalemia, symptomatic hypotension, allergic reactions, or angioedema), all patients with systolic and diastolic CHF should be maintained on an ACE inhibitor with or without a diuretic (Table 1.9).

ACE inhibitors are generally begun at low doses and titrated to the patient's blood pressure. Hypotension is reduced in patients who have adequate total body fluid; therefore diuretic doses may need to be lowered. Renal function should be monitored frequently (weekly to every 2 weeks) early in the course of therapy and periodically thereafter. Mild elevations of creatinine can occur without necessitating withdrawal of the medication.

Side Effects.   ACE inhibitors can produce hyperkalemia through their inhibition of aldosterone secretion. Electrolytes should be monitored and medication adjustments made if the serum potassium level becomes excessive. The concomitant use of potassium-sparing diuretics should be avoided. ACE inhibitor use is associated with maintenance of total-body potassium. Using potassium-sparing diuretics concomitantly may cause hyperkalemia. ACE inhibitors can cause renal insufficiency through altered renal blood flow. Severe renal insufficiency occurs in patients with renal artery stenosis. Renal function must be monitored in all patients receiving ACE inhibitors. These drugs should not be used in patients whose serum creatinine level exceeds 2.5 mg per dL, and they should be discontinued if the creatinine level doubles or exceeds 2.5 mg per dL with ACE inhibitor use.

Angiotensin 2 receptor blockers are associated with fewer toxicities, but improved survival studies are not completed.

Digoxin

Digoxin is an effective medication both to augment myocardial contractility and to suppress conduction through the AV node in patients with atrial fibrillation. These two actions are frequently referred to as the positive inotropic and negative chronotropic effects of digoxin.

Systolic CHF.   The clearest role for digoxin is in patients with systolic CHF who are in atrial fibrillation or who have supraventricular tachycardias. Digoxin will slow the ventricular response and improve contractility of the poorly functioning left ventricle.

The use of digoxin in patients with systolic dysfunction who are in normal sinus rhythm is controversial. Many such patients will show little or no response with the addition of digoxin to their treatment regimen. Digoxin should probably be reserved for use only if the patient has severe failure or is still symptomatic after employing a salt-restricted diet, using a diuretic, and receiving an appropriate dose of an ACE inhibitor. Dosing should start at 0.125 mg daily.

Diastolic CHF.   Digoxin should not be used in patients with diastolic CHF. The increased left ventricular contractility will cause increased left ventricular stiffness and decreased end-diastolic volume, causing an aggravation of the CHF.

Side Effects.   Digoxin has a narrow therapeutic window in the elderly, with a significant percentage of patients developing symptoms or signs of digoxin toxicity. Gastrointestinal toxicities such as anorexia and nausea can be insidious in the elderly and are easily blamed on other processes. Cardiotoxic manifestations with various heart blocks or arrhythmias are the most life-threatening complications.

Given the toxicity of digoxin, dosing in the elderly should be lower. Certainly, its dose for heart rate control should be adjusted only to achieve an adequate heart rate and should not be based on blood levels. For increasing contractility, most elderly patients will do well with doses of 0.125 mg per day. Only a few elderly patients need 0.25 mg per day, and higher doses should rarely be used.

Nitrates and Hydralazine

The combination of oral nitrates and hydralazine (Apresoline) provides for an excellent effect of decreased preload and afterload. It is useful in patients with both systolic and diastolic CHF. The main role of this combination is for patients in two situations:

- Those who cannot tolerate ACE inhibitors
- Those with continued symptoms who are receiving ACE inhibitors, diuretics, and digoxin

Dosing.   Oral nitrates are usually given as isosorbide dinitrate (Isorem) starting at a dose of 5 to 10 mg three times daily. This can be increased to a maximum of 40 mg three times daily. The dose of hydralazine is 25 mg and up to 100 mg three times a day. Lower doses may be appropriate in older patients with severe heart failure or hypotension.

Side Effects.   Both medications can cause hypotension and are usually titrated to the patient's blood pressure. Common side effects include headache and dizziness.

β-Blockers

Diastolic CHF.   The negative inotropic effect of β-blockers has made them a choice in the treatment of diastolic CHF. When the ventricular contractility is decreased, the filling of the ventricle is augmented and the CHF is improved. The negative chronotropic effects also allow for a longer diastole, thereby augmenting filling.

Another role for β-blockers is in patients with diastolic dysfunction who also have supraventricular tachycardias. Such patients' rates are better controlled with β-blockers and calcium channel blockers than with digoxin.

Systolic CHF.   The use of β-blockers in systolic CHF is a topic of great debate. For many years it was said that β-blockers were contraindicated in patients with CHF. However, this viewpoint has been questioned because of the data indicating a significant reduction in mortality in post–myocardial infarction (MI) patients receiving β-blockers, especially those who have CHF associated with MI. There are a number of studies indicating that patients with CHF without MI show benefits from β-blockers. Currently, the use of these drugs is not considered a standard of care, and β-blockers should not be given except when other modalities have been unsuccessful or when there is a specific indication for β-adrenergic blockade.

Dosing.   The dosing of β-blockers should initially be small, such as 10 mg of propranolol (Inderal) a day and titrated up gradually. Carvedilol (Coreg), a nonselective β-blocker with vasodilator effects, improves ventricular function in many patients. Careful titration is necessary to avoid worsening my-ocardial function through negative chronotropic and inotropic effects.

Calcium Channel Blockers

Diastolic CHF.   Calcium channel blockers have effects similar to those of β-blockers and are useful in patients with diastolic CHF. The negative inotropic and chronotropic effects allow for improved left ventricular filling. Nondihy-dropyridamole calcium channel blockers are best: verapamil (Calan), 40 to 120 mg every 8 hours; diltiazem (Cardizem), 30 to 90 mg every 6 hours.

Systolic CHF.   The older calcium channel blockers are still considered con-traindicated in patients with systolic CHF. The negative inotropic effects de-crease systolic contraction. Newer calcium channel blockers such as am-lodipine (Norvasc) or felodipine (Plendil) may be better choices because they are unassociated with an increase in symptoms or mortality.

Anticoagulants

Some authorities suggest that patients with severe systolic dysfunction (ejec-tion fraction less than 20 to 30%), especially those not in sinus rhythm, should receive oral anticoagulants to decrease the risk of cerebral embolization. Cer-tainly, patients with recent atrial fibrillation or a history of systemic or pul-monary embolism should receive anticoagulation.

Other Medications

At this time there are no other drugs that have been shown to benefit the ma-jority of patients with CHF. Other vasodilators have been tested, and none have been effective in decreasing symptoms or mortality like ACE inhibitors or nitrates and hydralazine. Oral phosphodiesterase inhibitors have been tried as potential agents to improve contractility without success. Outpatient intravenous dobutamine (Dobutrex) has been studied and found to be asso-ciated with increased mortality from ventricular arrhythmias. β-Adrenergic agonists have also been shown to increase mortality.

Other Treatment Modalities

Revascularization

Patients with CHF who have angina may be helped by coronary artery bypass surgery. Patients at high risk for silent ischemia may also benefit from this surgery. Revascularization in patients with CHF without evidence of is-chemia is more controversial.

FOLLOW-UP

The symptoms of CHF have classically been used to categorize the severity of disease. The New York Heart Association (NYHA) classification, which is widely used and accepted, is a useful way to document and follow symptom progression, despite its obvious subjectivity (Table 1.10).

- Close monitoring and follow-up clearly reduce hospitalization and improve the quality of life in patients with CHF.
- The most accurate measure of fluid status is vital signs, including body weight, and many physicians titrate diuretic doses to body weight.
- Continued diligence about medication and dietary compliance needs to be stressed.
- Patients taking diuretics need periodic blood testing for electrolytes.
- Digoxin level should be determined if appropriate.
- All CHF patients should have an annual ECG. Echocardiogram should be done periodically to assess status of ventricular function.
- Annual influenza vaccination and up-to-date vaccination for pneumococcus are important.
- As in all elderly patients, an advanced directive (a patient information sheet is included in the Appendix) should be completed by the patient in discussion with his or her family.

PATIENT EDUCATION

Patient education is essential in managing CHF (Table 1.11). A patient information sheet in included in the Appendix. Educational efforts should be positive and constructive. Compliance with drug therapy and dietary issues should be emphasized. A multidisciplinary program involving home nursing, nutritionists, and social workers, focusing on patient education with close outpatient monitoring, has been shown to lower rates of hospitalization and improve the quality of life. Patients should be taught how to recognize exacerbations.

TABLE 1.10. New York Heart Association (NYHA) Classification System for Heart Failure

Classification	Symptoms (i.e., fatigue, dyspnea)
Class I	No symptoms with normal activity; no limitation of physical activity
Class II	Symptoms of heart failure only with exercise; slight limitation to physical activity
Class III	Symptoms with mild exercise (e.g., walking), comfortable at rest; physical activity severely limited
Class IV	Symptoms at rest; incapable of any physical activity

TABLE 1.11. AHCPR Suggested Topics for Patient and Family Education

General counseling
Explanation of heart failure and the reason for symptoms
Cause or probable cause of the heart failure
Expected symptoms
Symptoms of worsening heart failure
What to do if symptoms worsen
Self-monitoring with daily weights
Explanation of treatment/care plan
Clarification of patient's responsibilities
Importance of cessation of tobacco use
Role of family members or other caregivers in the treatment/care plan
Availability and value of qualified local support group
Importance of obtaining vaccinations against influenza and pneumococcal disease

Prognosis
Life expectancy
Advance directives
Advice for family members in the event of sudden death

Activity recommendations
Recreation, leisure, and work activity
Exercise
Sex, sexual difficulties, and coping strategies

Dietary recommendations
Sodium restriction
Avoidance of excessive fluid intake
Fluid restriction (if required)
Alcohol restriction

Medications
Effects of medications on quality of life and survival
Dosing
Likely side effects and what to do if they occur
Coping mechanisms for complicated medical regimens
Availability of lower cost medications or financial assistance

Importance of compliance with the treatment/care plan

Reprinted from Konstam M, Dracup K, Baker D, et al. Heart failure: management of patients with left-ventricular systolic dysfunction. Quick reference guide for clinicians no. 11. AHCPR publication no. 94–0613. Rockville, MD: Agency for Health Care Policy and Research, Public Health Service, U.S. Dept. of Health and Human Services, 1994.

SUGGESTED READINGS

Aronow WS. Treatment of congestive heart failure in older persons. J Am Geriatr Soc 1997;45:1252-1257.

Konstam M, Dracup K, Baker D, et al. Heart failure: management of patients with left-ventricular systolic dysfunction. Quick reference guide for clinicians no. 11. AHCPR publication no. 94-0613. Rockville, MD: Agency for Health Care Policy and Research, Public Health Service, U.S. Dept. of Health and Human Services, 1994.

Mair FS. Management of heart failure. Am Fam Physician 1996;54:245-254.

Rich MW, Beckham V, Wittenberg C, et al. A multidisciplinary intervention to prevent the readmission of elderly patients with congestive heart failure. N Engl J Med 1995;333:1190-1195.

Senni M, Redfield MM. Congestive heart failure in elderly patients. Mayo Clin Proc 1997;72:453-460.

Senni M, Redfield MM. Congestive heart failure in the elderly. Mayo Clin Proc 1997;72:453-460.

Tresch DD, McGough MF. Heart failure with normal systolic function: a common disorder in older people. J Am Geriatr Soc 1995;43:1035-1042.

CHAPTER 2

Chronic Obstructive Pulmonary Disease

Chronic obstructive pulmonary disease (COPD) is the terminology for two disease states: chronic bronchitis and emphysema. The formal definition of chronic bronchitis is a productive cough that lasts for 3 months during two consecutive years. Emphysema, clinically characterized by obstruction to airflow, is defined pathologically as destruction of alveolar walls causing enlargement of distal air spaces. These conditions share a common characteristic—chronic limitation to expiratory airflow. Each has its own characteristic presentations and pathophysiology, but together they produce similar abnormalities in pulmonary function. In clinical practice the distinctions are rarely useful, especially as most patients with emphysema have components of chronic bronchitis as well. Some physicians will include asthma in the categorization of COPD, but pure bronchospastic asthma is rare in the elderly. Staging COPD by severity is helpful for prognosis and treatment planning (Table 2.1).

CHIEF COMPLAINT

Table 2.2 summarizes the common chief complaints of patients with chronic bronchitis or emphysema.

Chronic Bronchitis

Patients complain of a chronic cough, productive of sputum. The cough is daily and persistent, and the sputum can range from minimal clear mucus to a copious, purulent, discolored mucus when infection is present. Most patients will seek medical advice for the chronic cough and mucous production. Some patients may delay their need for care until they experience dyspnea with some mild exertion such as climbing stairs or walking up a hill.

TABLE 2.1.   American Thoracic Society Staging of COPD by Severity

Stage	Definition	Status
Stage I (Most patients)	$FEV_1 > 50\%$ of predicted value	Minimally affects quality of life
Stage II	FEV_1 35% to 49% of predicted value	Deterioration of quality of life
Stage III	$FEV_1 < 35\%$ of predicted value	Profound deterioration of quality of life

Adapted from Standards for the diagnosis and care of patients with chronic obstructive pulmonary disease. American Thoracic Society. Am J Respir Crit Care Med 1995;153:S77–121.
FEV_1 = forced expiratory volume in 1 second.

TABLE 2.2.   Clinical Presentation of Bronchitis and Emphysema

Clinical Presentation	Chronic Obstructive Bronchitis	Emphysema
Cough and sputum	Predominant symptom, frequently with copious and purulent sputum	Minimal and episodic
Dyspnea	Occurs early in the disease course, particularly with exertion	Onset is insidious, progressively worsens
Appearance (moderate/severe state)	Cyanotic, edematous, "blue bloater"	Cachetic, barrel-chested pursed lips, "pink puffer"

PATHOPHYSIOLOGY OF BRONCHITIS AND EMPHYSEMA

Chronic bronchitis is better termed chronic obstructive bronchitis, reflecting the underlying restriction to air flow. Pathologically, the lungs of patients with chronic obstructive bronchitis show airway mucosal inflammation, edema, and fibrosis with mucous gland hypertrophy. These underlying derangements are all reversible with appropriate therapies. The aging lung undergoes a loss of elasticity because of changes in collagen and a gradual loss of alveolar units, creating what some have called senile emphysema. However, without other insults, the lung has sufficient reserve to sustain function throughout a lifetime without any clinical symptoms. The term emphysema is used to describe the destruction of the alveolar walls and creation of large, air-space units within the lung. This creates a respiratory system that traps air, prevents normal expiratory forces, and impairs oxygen extraction within each air-space unit. Acute exacerbations can occur without a clear, precipitating cause, but are seen commonly with viral or bacterial lung infections. Other etiologies of acute exacerbations are atopic reactions with increased bronchial secretions and bronchospasm or other systemic illnesses that can affect pulmonary function such as abdominal illnesses or electrolyte disturbances. One important cause of an acute exacerbation of COPD is a spontaneous pneumothorax. The lungs of emphysematous patients, with the formation of large air pockets with thin walls (so-called blebs), are at risk for popping and creating a tension pneumothorax. In some patients this is a lethal event.

Emphysema

The patient usually complains of difficulty in breathing, and reports wheezing and the need to breath with pursed lips (creating a constant back-pressure of air to keep the airways open). Cough and sputum production are minimal. The patient usually presents with gradual progressive dyspnea.

Patients with COPD (both bronchitis or emphysema) are subject to periodic events of increased symptoms, referred to as acute exacerbations. Patients with these acute exacerbations present with rapidly developing dyspnea, tachypnea, tachycardia, and often a fever.

HISTORY

Disease-Stage Symptoms—Chronic Bronchitis

The patient may initially have no symptoms other than a slightly productive cough. The cough is usually worse at night and will lead to a loss of sleep, although the production of mucus is greatest on rising in the morning. Early in the course of the illness, the patient has symptoms limited to dyspnea with exertion. Sputum production is insidious, but worsens with time. Cough increases with time. As the disease progresses, the wheezing and dyspnea worsen, and the overexpansion of the pulmonary structure leads to the development of the barrel-like chest cavity. This produces a decline in the function of the respiratory muscles and will cause inadequate ventilation with a rising level of CO_2. With severe disease, there are frequent episodes of worsening airway obstruction from mucous blockade or airway inflammation, which cause acute hypoxemia and hypercapnia. Patients at this stage can also develop significant respiratory infections that lead to exacerbations. End stages of emphysema find a patient with significant hypoxia from any activity; with frequent admissions for exacerbations; and with progressive, hypercapneic respiratory failure. As the illness progresses, the cough and mucous production increases, infectious episodes set in, and dyspnea develops. Severe disease produces significant shortness of breath, excessive mucus,

---

EPIDEMIOLOGIC CONSIDERATIONS

COPD is closely associated with smoking, increasing age, childhood respiratory illnesses, environmental or occupational toxicities, and atopic disease. COPD occurs equally in elderly men and women, although the disease is more severe and the mortality is higher in men. COPD is the fourth leading cause of death in the elderly. There is a general consensus that COPD is underdiagnosed in the elderly because of the underutilization of pulmonary function tests (PFTs) and the relatively high prevalence of heart disease.

frequent infections, and the development of right-sided heart failure. Patients may lose weight.

A history of cigarette smoking is key to confirming the diagnosis. If the patient has no smoking history, the physician should search for a history of other toxins such as exposure to asbestos or silica or the presence of a genetic defect such as alpha 1 antitrypsin disease. There are some patients with pure bronchospastic asthma. The physician should obtain pertinent medical history, including information about other concomitant illnesses, hematologic disorders, heart disease, and all medications. An assessment of the impact of the patients' symptoms on their functional status is crucial.

PHYSICAL EXAMINATION

The physical examination of the chest will aid in confirming the diagnosis of COPD. Early in the disease the physician may find some subtle changes of the loss of alveolar air-space units and obstruction to airflow. These early findings include tachypnea, decreased breath sounds, hyperresonance of the chest, and flattening of the diaphragm with displacement of the heart's point of maximal impulse (PMI) inferiorly and laterally. Coarse crackles may be heard at the lung bases. As the disease progresses, the chest will take on a barrel shape, and the patient will start to purse his or her lips and use accessory muscles to aid in respirations. Wheezing can frequently be heard on chest auscultation, usually on expiration first, and later on both inspiration and expiration. Right-sided heart failure, with distension of the jugular veins, hepatic congestion, and peripheral edema, occurs late in the disease as the pulmonary arterial resistance increases.

DIAGNOSTIC TEST DATA

Diagnostic testing is essential to the diagnosis and management of COPD. Pulmonary function testing (PFT) is mandatory in all patients with COPD, as well as any patient in whom the diagnosis is suspected, to detect the presence and reversibility of airflow obstruction. Arterial blood gases (ABGs) and plain chest films are necessary in certain circumstances, for example, acute exacerbations and acute dyspnea.

Pulmonary Function Tests (PFTs)

The PFT is the diagnostic test of choice in situations in which the diagnosis is uncertain. PFTs should be performed at the time of initial presentation and periodically throughout the care of COPD patients. PFTs can be done with an office-based spirometer, which gives at least a FEV_1 (forced expiratory volume in 1 second) and an FVC (forced vital capacity). Spirometry in patients with undiseased, aged lungs shows increased functional residual capacity and residual volume without an increase in total lung capacity. The FEV_1 gradually declines, as does the normal level of measured PaO_2 (estimated by the formula $100 - 1/3 \times$ age in years). The FEV_1 is interpreted against predicted values and can also be analyzed in a ratio to the FVC. An FEV_1:FVC ratio should be greater than 0.8; if it is less than 0.7, it clearly confirms the diagnosis of COPD. Symptoms of dyspnea usually begin when the FEV_1 falls below 60% of predicted values, and end-stage disease is reflected when the FEV_1 falls to 20%. PFTs should be performed annually to determine disease progression. They are also useful during exacerbations to determine illness severity and effects of treatment. More sophisticated testing can measure other pulmonary functions and give some further details such as diffuse capacity, minute ventilation, and effect of bronchodilators on lung functions. These details may be helpful in difficult cases or when the diagnosis is questioned. Office-based testing is most often sufficient.

Arterial Blood Gases (ABGs)

ABGs are not necessary to make or confirm a diagnosis of COPD. ABGs should be obtained when a patient's dyspnea begins to limit activities (stage II or stage III). ABGs are essential in evaluating acute exacerbations of COPD. They are also a requirement for determining a patient's need for chronic oxygen therapy. ABGs are used in patients with moderate to severe dyspnea. Because of their impaired ventilation, COPD patients will have elevations of carbon dioxide on their ABGs leading to chronic respiratory acidosis. Their pH is normal in their usual state because of compensation for their acidosis by retention of renal bicarbonate (serum HCO_3 of 30 to 40). Their PO_2 is usually depressed in their baseline state. So a typical ABG in a patient with moderate COPD in their usual state will show a pH of 7.35 to 7.40, a PCO_2 of 40 to 50, and a PO_2 of 55 to 70. During an exacerbation, or as the patient's disease progresses, the ABGs worsen to reflect a chronic acidosis of <7.35, an increase in PCO_2 (typically in the 50s), and a reduced PO_2 (50s).

Plain Chest Films

Plain films play a limited role in disease diagnosis and management. It is well known that they show little about actual pulmonary function and correlate poorly with symptoms in COPD. The chest film of a patient with COPD is abnormal with pulmonary hyperinflation, flattening of the diaphragm, and a narrow cardiac silhouette. The presence of blebs is important in indicating a risk for development of a pneumothorax. The physician should obtain a plain chest film during acute exacerbations to look for pneumothorax or pneumonia. Chest films do have a role in ruling out other important pulmonary diseases such as acute or chronic infections (e.g., tuberculosis) or lung cancer. (See Table 2.3 for differential diagnosis.)

TABLE 2.3. Differential Diagnosis of COPD

Differential Diagnosis	Distinguishing Characteristics
Acute viral or bacterial infection	Acute-onset fever, systemic symptoms, myalgias, fatigue
Chronic infections: tuberculosis, fungal, etc.	Focal findings on chest film; fever; lack of hypercapnia
Pulmonary tumor or metastatic disease	Focal findings on chest film, lack of hypercapnia and hypoxemia, weight loss prominent early in disease
Congestive heart failure	Systemic evidence of fluid retention, pulmonary rales, chest film shows fluid, jugular venous distension
Sarcoidosis	Occurs rarely among elderly, pulmonary nodules or hilar adenopathy on chest film, hypercalcemia
Pulmonary embolism	Acute-onset, prominent tachycardia; hypoxemia without hypercapnia; chest film normal or with mild atelectasis
Pulmonary hypertension	Rare among the elderly, normal chest film, lack of hypercapnia
Interstitial lung diseases, pulmonary fibrosis, rheumatoid lung, drug or occupationally induced lung disease	Chest film shows abnormal interstitial markings; pulmonary functions are restrictive not obstructive; history of rheumatic disease or occupational exposure

Pulse Oximetry

Pulse oximetry provides physicians with a noninvasive tool to monitor oxygen saturations. This is very useful in monitoring the status of disease during acute exacerbations. However, the pulse oximeter cannot determine the level of PCO_2 or acidosis and therefore cannot replace the ABG in managing COPD patients.

Electrocardiogram

Electrocardiograms (ECGs) are important in the ongoing management of patients and are certainly indicated in evaluating and managing acute exacerbations.

Other Tests

Blood work (Mg levels, phosphate levels, CBCs, and creatinine) is important in ongoing management and acute exacerbations because of potential derangements caused by metabolic or infectious processes. If pulmonary infection causes an acute exacerbation, sputum cultures should be done to determine the most predominant organism. They have no role in the chronic management of COPD.

DIFFERENTIAL DIAGNOSIS

Although other diseases can produce symptoms similar to COPD (Table 2.3), the older patient presenting to the family physician's office with complaints of gradual progressive dyspnea, chronic cough, or chronic sputum production should raise the possibility of COPD. The history, physical, and laboratory findings can confirm this diagnosis. The patient will give a history of smoking and will have some physical findings showing, at a minimum, decreased breath sounds, mild expiratory wheezing, and hyperresonance of the chest cavity. Office spirometry will show a FEV_1 that is 60% of that predicted or a FEV_1:FVC ratio of 0.7, which is all that is necessary to diagnose COPD and to plan therapy.

Although the distinctions between chronic bronchitis and emphysema are interesting, they are rarely clinically helpful. The vast majority of patients have a clinical picture of emphysema associated with a component of chronic bronchitis to their illness. For that reason most authors and clinicians unify these two diseases and refer to them as COPD.

WHEN TO REFER

The referral of patients with COPD to pulmonary specialists is usually unnecessary. The management of early disease, acute exacerbations, and progressive illness can be handled by the family physician. As in any illness, the family physician who is uncomfortable with particular situations should always consider appropriate consultation or referral. Comprehensive pulmonary rehabilitation programs are important resources for the patient with COPD. Such services should be considered for all patients as their disease progresses.

MANAGEMENT

A general approach to the management of COPD is shown in Figure 2.1.

Pharmacologic

A number of medications have been used for COPD. The direct action of medications within the pulmonary tree has become the mainstay of COPD therapy, with aerosolized preparations delivered via a system called a metered-dose inhaler (MDI). Table 2.4 summarizes drugs available in this formulation.

Optimizing the Use of Inhalers

Metered-dose inhalers (MDIs) are the mainstay of therapy for COPD. However, their use is not simple, and many patients are unable to optimize therapy

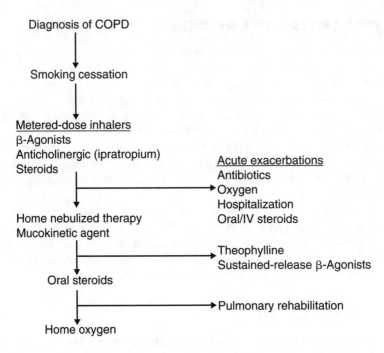

Diagnosis of COPD

Smoking cessation

Metered-dose inhalers
β-Agonists
Anticholinergic (ipratropium)
Steroids

Acute exacerbations
Antibiotics
Oxygen
Hospitalization
Oral/IV steroids

Home nebulized therapy
Mucokinetic agent

Theophylline
Sustained-release β-Agonists

Oral steroids

Pulmonary rehabilitation

Home oxygen

FIGURE 2.1. Treatment flowchart for chronic obstructive pulmonary disease (COPD).

because of the mechanics involved in using MDIs. The following guidelines are given to optimize the efficacy of MDIs for the elderly:

- Ensure that the patient is not limited by cognitive ability or severe arthritis.
- Prescribe a spacer with all MDIs.
- Demonstrate appropriate MDI use as follows:
  - Start inhalation immediately from end of exhalation.
  - Activate MDI just after start of inhalation.
  - Inhale slowly.
  - Hold breath after inhalation for 10 seconds.
  - Repeat to obtain two actuations during one treatment.
- Observe the patient performing the above steps.
- Reeducate the patient about appropriate techniques at follow-up visits.

MDIs require some strength and coordination to use appropriately, and this may pose a problem in certain elderly patients. Spacers are available that have improved therapy with MDIs by decreasing the droplet size and slowing the particle velocity.

Other Drugs

Theophylline is a weak bronchodilator and acts to strengthen the diaphragm, thereby decreasing the severity of dyspnea in patients with COPD. In the elderly the toxicity (tremor, tachycardia, nausea, and anxiety) and drug interactions (warfarin [Coumadin], selective serotonin reuptake inhibitors) limit its use to the rare patient. Theophylline blood levels must be followed closely if this agent is chosen, and target serum levels are lower than usual (5 to 15 μg per mL).

Antibiotics are commonly used in the treatment of patients with COPD. Recurrent pulmonary infections are frequent in patients with both chronic bronchitis and emphysema. Antibiotics should be initiated early in the infections to decrease morbidity, and it is prudent to provide patients with broad-spectrum, oral antibiotics for home use when a change in sputum or fever is noted. The most common pathogens are *Streptococcus pneumoniae, Haemophilus influenzae,* and *Moraxella catarrhalis.* Antibiotics such as tetracyclines, second-generation cephalosporins, macrolides, azilides, trimethoprim/sulfamethoxazole (Bactrim), and amoxicillin/clavulanate (Augmentin) are effective. Long-term antibiotic use to suppress infections has not been demonstrated to be of benefit.

TABLE 2.4.   Medications Administered Via Metered-Dose Inhalers[a] for the Treatment of COPD

Drug Class	Mechanism of Action	Common Agents	Comments
β-Adrenergic agonists	Bronchodilation via direct, smooth-muscle relaxation	Albuterol (Ventolin); bitolterol (Tornalate); metaproterenol (Alupent); pirbuterol (Maxair); salmeterol (Serevent)	Short acting. Dosing: two puffs, four to six times per day Long acting. Dosing: two puffs, one to two times per day
Anticholinergics	Large, bronchial dilation via cholinergic receptors on smooth muscle	Ipratropium (Atrovent)	MDI delivery system alone or mixed with β-agonist; two puffs, four to six times per day
Anti-inflammatories	Decrease airway edema and secretions; stabilize mast cells	Corticosteroids	MDIs best; can be given orally; parentally for acute exacerbations
		Cromolyn (Intal)	MDIs only
		Nedocromil (Tilade)	MDIs only

aUseful combination inhalers are available to improve patient convenience and compliance.

Other Treatment Modalities

Smoking Cessation

For patients with early disease, the underlying pathology can be reversed almost entirely if smoking is discontinued. If the disease is allowed to progress, the underlying damage to lung tissue becomes irreversible. Even in these patients, however, smoking cessation is beneficial and slows progression of the illness. The oxygen-dependent patient should not be smoking. Smoking cessation will also lessen the risk of heart disease, stroke, peripheral vascular disease, and osteoporosis. Smoking cessation should be emphasized in patients with COPD. Below is a list of some specific steps for the family physician to take to help patients stop smoking:

- Explicitly advise the patient to stop smoking.
- Establish a contract with the patient that includes a stop date.
- Assist the patient with nicotine replacement and withdrawal.
- Use printed, self-help materials and direct the patient to a formal, smoking-cessation program.
- Continue to educate and encourage the patient to stop smoking.

Immunizations

Patients with COPD should receive annual influenza vaccinations. These are available each autumn and are recommended to be given as a single injection during late October/early November. Pneumococcal multivalent vaccine is also standard for patients with COPD. One single vaccination is effective for a lifetime in most situations. There have been recommendations to reimmunize individuals vaccinated more than 6 years previously who (1) were less than 65 years of age at first vaccination or (2) are debilitated from diabetes, heart disease, renal disease, liver disease, or pulmonary disease. Therefore, revaccinate if (1) the patient received the first vaccine at age 65 or less, and if it is now 6 years or more since the first vaccine; or (2) the patient received the first vaccine 6 years or more ago and is debilitated from diabetes, heart, renal, liver, or pulmonary disease.

Home Oxygen Therapy

Supplemental oxygen can decrease pulmonary hypertension, reduce secondary polycythemia, improve neuropsychiatric function, and decrease breathlessness. Overall functional abilities are improved, as is the patient's quality of life. Oxygen therapy can be detrimental, however, if not used carefully. Excess supplemental oxygen will reduce respiratory drive and lead to CO_2 retention, respiratory acidosis, and a gradual decline of mental function that, in turn, will lead to coma and death. ABGs must be obtained to ensure appropriate oxygen administration. Oxygen is administered in continuous flow by nasal cannula at the lowest liter flow rate needed to bring the PO_2 to 60 to 65 mm Hg or the oxygen saturation to 88 to 94%. The baseline

TABLE 2.5. Oxygen Delivery Systems in Treatment of COPD

System	Characteristics	Comments
Stationary	Large reservoirs or oxygen-producing devices (gas cylinders, liquid reservoirs, or oxygen concentrators)	Gas cylinders or liquid reservoirs contain 1-month supplies and can be used to refill ambulatory systems. Oxygen concentrators do not require refilling; other systems cannot be refilled
Portable	Small oxygen cylinders or concentrators mounted on a cart	Poor choice in ambulatory patients; limits mobility. Useful for transporting patients
Ambulatory	Oxygen in gas or liquid form in 5.5-lb, strap-on canisters. Four hours of oxygen available	Refillable canisters; useful for performing duties around the house and on short trips

liter flow rate should be increased by 1 liter during exercise and sleep. Medicare reimbursement is available for home oxygen supplementation if the patient meets eligibility standards (room air PaO_2 of <55 or from 55 to 59 with evidence of polycythemia, pulmonary hypertension, or right-sided heart failure). Types of oxygen-delivery systems are listed in Table 2.5.

Pulmonary Rehabilitation

Comprehensive pulmonary rehabilitation services include physiotherapy for muscle training and reconditioning, psychotherapy, patient and family education, and occupational therapy for work simplification and energy conservation. Smoking cessation programs are commonly included in these programs. Many communities have successful programs for patients with moderate to severe COPD.

FOLLOW-UP

Monitoring Disease Course

The patient with COPD requires a close relationship with the physician to monitor and manage this chronic disease.

Some measure of pulmonary function, either with peak flow measurements or simple spirometry, should be obtained, as a routine, one to three times a year to document disease progression.

Annual immunizations should be administered. In addition, visits every 2 to 3 months for patients with moderate to severe disease can focus on compliance with and effectiveness of medications, psychosocial support, and patient education.

The last phases of COPD create significant anxiety as episodes of breathlessness increase. Management requires careful anxiolysis and judicious morphine use to decrease the dyspnea. Increasing the oral steroid dose to 40 to 60 mg a day of prednisone should be considered to maximize anti-inflammatory effects, increase appetite, and create a mild euphoria associated with steroids. Managing the terminal phase of end-stage COPD requires physician diligence. Patients need a clear, durable power of attorney, as they are at high risk of needing ventilatory support and thereby may be unable to communicate their wishes effectively.

PATIENT EDUCATION

The following are key areas to cover with patients:

- That smoking cessation is primary
- That exercise maintains cardiovascular conditioning
  - Aerobic exercises for conditioning (e.g., bicycling, walking, swimming)
  - Resistance exercises for strengthening knee, hip, shoulders (weightlifting)
  - Stretching exercises for flexibility
- Proper use of MDIs and spacers
- Early recognition of acute exacerbations and instituting increased steroids, antibiotics, increased nebulized medications
- Diet: increased nutrition—add liquid protein, caloric supplements
- To watch for symptoms/signs of depression
- Airplane travel: may need supplemental oxygen if predicted O_2 saturation is <90
- That supplemental oxygen is useful during periods of breathlessness, but flow rate must be kept below 2 L per minute
- That antibiotics may be useful at the first sign of an acute exacerbation

SUGGESTED READINGS

Daniels S, Meuleman J. Importance of assessment of metered-dose inhaler technique in the elderly. J Am Geriatr Soc 1994;42:82–84.

Dosman JA, Cockcroft DW, eds. Obstructive lung disease. Medical Clinics of North America, WB Saunders, 1990.

Holleman DR, Simel DL, Goldberg JS, et al. Diagnosis of obstructive airways disease from the clinical examination. J Gen Intern Med 1993;8:63–68.

Rimer BK, Orleans CT, Resch N, et al. The older smokers: status, challenges and opportunities for intervention. Chest 1990;97:547–553.

CHAPTER 3

··

Dementia

MANIFESTATIONS

Dementia, or cognitive decline, is not a normal part of aging. It is a disorder that can go unrecognized, as it has a slow, gradual progression that is frequently mistaken for simply "growing old." Dementia is defined as an acquired persistent impairment in intellectual function that affects three or more of the following areas:

• Memory
• Emotions/personality
• Visual-spatial skills
• Language
• Cognition (calculation, intelligence, judgment)

It is estimated to affect 10% of individuals over age 65, 20% of individuals from age 75 to 84, and almost 50% of seniors over age 85.

Memory

The characteristic memory change is a loss in the most recent short-term memory centers. Memory for remote events is usually well preserved, although defects in remote recall are also noted as the disease progresses. Learning is severely affected, with a progressive inability to acquire any new factual information.

Disorientation to time and place are early findings in demented individuals. Patients will frequently forget commonplace household routines that require short-term memory such as turning off lights or running water, closing doors, or flushing toilets.

Emotions/Personality

Demented patients seem to withdraw from work or family events and tend to place less importance on socialization. Casual conversation is maintained, although the content of the conversation is more general, with few specific details. Language tends to be fluid, sometimes loquacious, and phrases or cliches are overutilized.

Frequently, family members report personality change. Demented individuals are described as more apathetic, especially in their approach to dress or hygiene. Occasionally, the patient will show less control of impulses, with outbursts of anger or inappropriate foul language. Frank delusions or hallucinations are uncommon until late in the disease. Demented patients usually will not attempt to explain or compensate for these changes, as they do not recognize them as alterations from their normal behavior.

Visual-Spatial Skills

Disruption of visual-spatial orientation can cause a person with dementia to get lost in familiar surroundings or become unable to use tools, instruments, or cooking utensils. Also, an impairment in dressing ("dressing apraxia"), buttoning shirts, or tying shoes often occurs.

Language

Patients with dementia have a language disturbance characterized by a difficulty in finding the correct word for an item. This is not a true aphasia, in which the word is known but unable to be expressed, but more an anomia, in which the word cannot be located in the memory. The demented person frequently can describe the use of an object, or demonstrate its use, but cannot find the correct name for it. Spouses may unintentionally cover up the demented person's language or memory errors by answering questions or completing sentences for the person.

Cognition

Cognitive impairment is relative to the individual's prior intellectual abilities. Most individuals have a loss in the ability to do simple mathematics or spelling. Highly intelligent individuals with extensive vocabularies may retain the ability to do simple subtraction or spelling, showing abnormalities only if tested for complex mathematical or verbal skills. Cognitive function decline

AGE-ASSOCIATED MEMORY IMPAIRMENT (AAMI)

AAMI is a commonly cited disorder that is felt to represent a normal age-related decline in memory. The distinction between age-associated memory impairment and dementia is that memory impairment is a nonprogressive loss that has little effect on an individual's functional abilities. AAMI typically affects the following: (1) memory for names of people, especially new acquaintances, and (2) recent minor events such as where the car keys were last left.

can be lessened through continued use of intellectual stimuli such as solving crossword puzzles or reading.

CHIEF COMPLAINT

Patients with true dementia are commonly brought to a physician by their family or caregivers, as they are unaware or deny the significance of their cognitive disturbance. In fact, patients who see a physician of their own volition with a concern about memory loss or cognitive decline more commonly have depression rather than dementia.

HISTORY

The most useful information is obtained from family, friends, or caregivers, and not from the patients themselves, even early in the disease. The historical clues that aid in the differential diagnosis relate to the following:

Onset/Duration of Symptoms

- Symptoms that have come on over more than 6 months and have been slowly progressive are typical for patients with Alzheimer's disease.
- A stepwise deterioration, with plateaus and acute deterioration to a new level, is characteristic of a multiple infarct dementia syndrome.
- A more acute onset—days to weeks—is indicative of a potentially treatable cause of the dementia such as a drug-induced state, thyroid disease, or subdural hematoma. Sudden onset of mental status changes are more commonly caused by delirium (Table 3.1).
- A recent history of head trauma, followed by a decline in mental function— it is important to rule out subdural hematoma.

Other Symptoms

- Dementia from an organic brain lesion such as a subdural hematoma, brain tumor, or normal pressure hydrocephalus almost always presents with such neurologic symptoms as weakness and gait and visual ataxias, in addition to the dementia.
- Neuromuscular or neurosensory losses, urinary incontinence, severe headaches, or gait disturbances can lead a physician to the underlying dementing process.

Medication Use

- Medication-induced brain dysfunction is exceptionally common in older adults; potential offending agents such as anticholinergics, sedatives, and hypnotics should be stopped.

TABLE 3.1.   **Signs of Delirium and Dementia**

Signs	Delirium	Dementia
Onset	Sudden	Slow
Daily course	Fluctuating, with nocturnal exacerbations	Stable
Consciousness	Reduced	Clear
Attention	Disordered	Normal, except in severe cases
Cognition	Disordered	Impaired
Orientation	Usually impaired, at least for a time	Frequently impaired
Psychomotor activity	Increased, reduced or changing erratically	Often normal
Speech	Often incoherent, slow or rapid	Patient has difficulty finding words, perseveration in severe disease state
Involuntary movements	Often asterixis or coarse tremor	Usually absent
Physical illness or drug toxicity	One or both are present	Often absent, especially in senile dementia of the Alzheimer type

Adapted from Bross MH, Tatum NO. Delirium in the elderly patient. Am Fam Physician 1994;50(6):1325–1332.

- The abrupt withdrawal of certain drugs, particularly alcohol or benzodi-azepines, can cause mental status changes.

PHYSICAL EXAMINATION

General Physical Status

As many systems can be related to dementia, a comprehensive physical exam should always be performed.

- The neurologic exam must include an evaluation of the patient's gait, as well as his or her neuromuscular and neurosensory status.
- The ophthalmologic exam is critical. Papilledema, indicating elevations in CNS pressure, can be found in subdural hematomas or brain tumors. The testing of visual fields by confrontation is important; the visual cortical connections occupy a large area of the brain.

Mental-Status Testing

The key to diagnosing dementia is the mental status. All seniors should undergo screening for cognitive function. Patients identified by screening should undergo formal, mental-status testing.

Screening

Although many practicing physicians find the 12-item, 30-point, Mini-Mental Status Exam (MMSE) too time consuming to use as a screening test, the three questions below can be used as a screening tool for all seniors:

- Orientation: Ask the person the day, date, year, and current location.
- Registration/recall: Name three new objects and ask the individual to repeat them immediately and to recall them after 3 to 5 minutes.
- Cognitive function: Ask the individual to subtract serial 7s from 100 or to spell a word (e.g., WORLD) backwards.

Any patient who performs poorly in these three areas should complete the entire MMSE.

Formal Testing

The MMSE may be administered by any health care provider. It is highly accurate in identifying individuals with dementia. Those without the disorder will score a minimum of 27; those with dementia typically score under 24. Subjects who score between 24 and 27 are more likely than normal individuals to show a decline on repeat testing. A copy of the MMSE is provided in the Appendix.

Tracking Progression

The clock-drawing test is useful for tracking the progression of dementia. Ask the patient to draw the face of a clock, place the numbers appropriately, and include the clock hands at a specified time (e.g., 1:45).

DIAGNOSTIC TEST DATA

The use of diagnostic testing in the evaluation of dementia has been overemphasized in the past 10 years. The treatable causes of dementia, once thought to represent 15 to 20% of all dementias, probably represent less than 5% of cases, and the majority of these cases are identified by a thorough history and a physical exam. However, the following laboratory and radiographic tests are considered standard by many.

- Complete blood cell count (CBC)—Screening for anemia, macrocytosis, or hypersegmented polymorphonuclear cells to suggest B_{12} deficiency or leukocytosis to suggest infection
- Electrolytes/glucose—For hyper- or hyponatremia, hyper- or hypoglycemia, and elevated creatinine, suggestive of renal insufficiency
- Calcium—For hypercalcemia, suggestive of metastatic disease or hyperparathyroidism
- Liver function tests—For liver failure, findings suggesting alcoholism, or hepatic/biliary tumors

- Thyroid testing—For hyper- or hypothyroidism
- Human immunodeficiency virus (HIV) testing—For evidence of acquired immunodeficiency syndrome (AIDS) dementia or HIV-associated diseases
- VDR—For neurosyphilis
- Electrocardiogram (ECG)—For ischemia, arrhythmias such as atrial fibrillation or bradycardias, or evidence of heart failure
- Urinalysis—For infection
- Chest film—For malignancies or signs of active tuberculosis
- Computed tomographic (CT) scan—For tumor, normal pressure hydrocephalus, or subdural hematomas

Other optional studies may include the following:

- Electroencephalogram (EEG)—If seizures are suspected
- Lumbar puncture—If meningitis is suspected

DIFFERENTIAL DIAGNOSIS

An excellent resource is the Agency for Health Care Policy and Research's clinical practice guidelines on Recognition and Initial Assessment of Alzheimer's Disease and Related Dementias.

Alzheimer's Disease

Although it is not possible to make a definitive diagnosis of Alzheimer's disease without a brain biopsy or autopsy, the following clinical criteria are reasonably accurate:

- Dementing illness confirmed by mental status testing with deficits in two or more areas of cognition
- Onset between age 40 and 90; most commonly around 65
- No disturbance of consciousness
- Progressive worsening in memory and cognitive function
- Absence of brain or systemic disorders that could account for the progressive brain dysfunction

Multiple-Infarct Dementia

Multiple-infarct dementia results from an accumulation of lacunar infarcts in the cortical and/or subcortical areas of the brain, which occur as a result of occlusion of the most distal vessels of arterial circulation that have no collateral circulation. Affected areas tend to be in the temporal/parietal lobes in areas responsible for memory and cognitive function. CT scan may or may not show evidence of these or other infarcts, as they result in such small areas of necrotic brain. The clinical picture is frequently identical to that of patients with Alzheimer's disease, with the following exceptions:

- Patients have a stepwise deterioration with plateaus. Each step is abrupt in onset and presents as a sudden worsening of the clinical picture.
- Patients frequently have focal, neurologic signs and symptoms (hemisensory or hemimotor loss). Other, more subtle focal neurologic signs include gait disturbance, positive Babinski's sign and asymmetric reflexes.
- Patients commonly have a history of hypertension, smoking, atherosclerotic disease, and stroke.

Normal-Pressure Hydrocephalus

Normal-pressure hydrocephalus accounts for less than 1% of all cases of dementias. It is an idiopathic disorder that results in dilation of the cerebrospinal fluid ventricular system, which damages the cortical tissue. CT scan shows characteristic changes that include dilation of the ventricular system with flattening of the cerebral sulci. The dementia caused by normal-pressure hydrocephalus is clinically identical to that of Alzheimer's disease or multiple-infarct dementia. However, the following clinical triad is the hallmark of this diagnosis:

- Dementia
- Urinary incontinence
- Gait disorder (an apraxia that looks as if the feet are magnetized to the floor)

Creutzfeld-Jakob Disease

Creutzfeld-Jakob disease results from a slow virus infection of the brain. It can be transmitted by ingestion or transplantation of infected tissue. The dementia is distinguished from that of Alzheimer's disease as follows:

- The victims are generally younger.
- The condition is more rapidly progressive.
- Associated neurologic abnormalities such as myoclonic jerks, severe rigidity, and asymmetric reflex findings exist.
- An EEG shows characteristic high-voltage bursts of bi- and triphasic slow waves.

Dementias Associated with Other Neurologic Disorders

Memory and cognitive dysfunction is seen as part of other neurologic diseases such as Parkinson's disease, Huntington's disease, or Down syndrome. Patients with these diseases usually have prominent symptoms of their disease and mild dementia symptoms. A patient with Parkinson's disease and dementia has prominent parkinsonian features—tremor, rigidity, cogwheeling, change in facies, micrographia, gait changes—and mild cognitive dysfunction. Patients with Huntington's disease have prominent chorea and mild dementia. For patients with Down syndrome, cognitive and/or memory loss is not present at birth, but develops later in life.

Potentially Reversible Causes of Dementia

The mnemonic DEMENTIA is used to categorize the potentially reversible causes of dementia:

D = Drugs
E = Emotional disorders
M = Metabolic or endocrine disorders
E = Eye and ear disorders
N = Nutritional deficiencies
T = Tumor or trauma
I = Infections
A = Arteriosclerotic complications such as myocardial infarction or congestive heart failure and alcohol

The screening tests described above are designed to detect these potentially reversible causes. However, the detection of these causes does not guarantee that the dementia can or will be reversed with treatment.

WHEN TO REFER

Because dementia is typically a progressive disease that requires a coordination of services, it is important to stay intimately involved in the patient's care. Additional resources in the evaluation of management of demented patients include the following:

- Consultation with a neurologist may be beneficial if the patient presents with atypical findings.
- Referral for more advanced neuropsychologic testing if unusual findings occur on mental-status testing.
- Care facilities that specialize in patients with dementia, in coordination with the family physician.
- If diagnostic tests hint at potentially treatable causes, consultation with the appropriate subspecialist may be useful.

MANAGEMENT

Management of the patient with dementia focuses on three areas:

- Treatment of the decline in memory and cognition
- Treatment of behavioral problems
- Overall approach to the patient as it relates to his/her dementia

Treatment of Decline in Memory and Cognition

Cholinesterase Inhibitors

The underlying pathology of memory and cognitive decline appears to be structural loss of neurons with a depletion of the neurochemical acetylcholine. Replacement of acetylcholine, through the use of an acetylcholinesterase inhibitor, has been shown to improve memory and cognitive function in patients with mild dementia and to delay progression of the disease by approximately 6 months. Two drugs, tacrine (Cognex) and donepezil (Aricept), are currently available.

Tacrine has significant limitations to its use:

- It is hepatotoxic, particularly at the effective dose of 160 mg per day.
- It interacts with medications metabolized by the cytochrome p450 system of the liver such as benzodiazepines, H2 blockers, and theophylline.
- It is poorly absorbed if taken with food.
- It induces nausea and vomiting in up to 25% of patients.

Given all of these issues, tacrine has found limited use in the treatment of dementia by most primary care physicians.

The new cholinesterase inhibitor, donepezil, was approved in the winter of 1997. Donepezil has several potential advantages compared with tacrine:

- It is less hepatotoxic.
- It can be given once a day.
- It does not interfere with liver metabolism.
- It can be given with food
- It appears to have equal efficacy to tacrine.

Estrogen

Estrogen is the only other medication to have an impact on memory and cognitive function. Several retrospective studies have demonstrated that fewer women on estrogen replacement developed Alzheimer's disease. In addition, nonrandomized studies of estrogen use show that patients with Alzheimer's disease experience improvement in global measures of cognitive function. However, because of a lack of a sufficient number of studies, the evidence is suspect at this point; a current prospective randomized trial should provide more solid data about the role of estrogen in therapy for memory and cognitive decline.

Other Agents

Other agents that have been tried to improve cognitive function or prevent cognitive decline include nonsteroidal anti-inflammatory drugs; botanical agents such as ginkgo biloba; selegiline; and vitamin E. The evidence of clinical benefit from any of these agents is inconclusive. At this time the use of these agents should be limited to experimental protocols only.

Treatment of Behavioral Problems

Demented patients display many behavioral problems as their cognitive function declines. Behavioral problems may include the following:

- Wandering
- Aggression
- Incontinence
- Repetitive episodes of inappropriate shouting
- Insomnia
- Public displays of sexual behavior

Therapy for behavioral problems should begin with anticipatory guidance. Behavioral modifications alone may control some distressing or dangerous behaviors. Some of these modifications include the following:

- Create a safe environment for a wandering patient by placing complex opening mechanisms on certain doors, hiding car keys, or placing protective devices on kitchen stoves and ovens.
- Aid the patient with scheduled voidings to manage incontinence.
- Avoid disorienting situations such as new environments or extreme darkness.

Drug therapy for behavioral problems in demented patients is nonspecific and centers around various sedative medications. In general, antipsychotic neuroleptics, sedative/hypnotics, and antidepressants are most commonly used.

Neuroleptics

All of the phenothiazine-type neuroleptics are efficacious in the treatment of delusions, hallucinations, and aggressive behaviors. Haloperidol (Haldol) and risperidone (Risperdal) are highly potent; thioridazine and chlorpromazine are low potency. Potency is inversely related to the risk of extrapyramidal side effects such as tardive dyskinesias and parkinsonism. High-potency medications are the most likely to cause these movement disorders. Table 3.2 summarizes these medications.

Sedatives/Hypnotics

Benzodiazepines have been the drug of choice for the treatment of anxiety in demented individuals, but have also been useful in the management of insomnia and, occasionally, agitation. Metabolism of the benzodiazepines is slowed in the elderly, and they can accumulate and cause excessive sedation and worsening cognitive function.

TABLE 3.2. Neuroleptics for the Treatment of Behavioral Problems in Patients with Dementia

Medication	Dosage (per day)	Potency	Sedation	Anticholinergic Effects	Side Effects
Haloperidol (Haldol)	0.5 to 10 mg	High	+	+	Tardive dyskinesia, Parkinsonism
Risperidone (Risperdal)	0.25 to 3 mg	High	+	+	Dyskinesias and hypotension
Thioridazine (Mellaril)	10 to 200 mg	Low	+++	++	Quinidine-like effects on the heart
Chlorpromazine (Thorazine)	10 to 100 mg	Low	+++	+++	Hypotension and seizures
Clozapine (Clozaril)	12.5 to 200 mg	Low	+++	+++	Agranulocytosis

The short half-life drugs such as lorazepam (Ativan) and alprazolam (Xanax) are preferred. The adage "start low and go slow" should be used in prescribing benzodiazepines. Continuous use is best avoided because of addictive potential and withdrawal seizures.

Buspirone (Buspar), an anxiolytic unrelated to the benzodiazepines, has been used to treat agitation with perhaps less sedation than other drugs used for anxiety.

Antidepressants

Used in the therapy of depression in demented individuals (see Chapter 4 on depression), these drugs are also useful in the treatment of agitation and insomnia. The least anticholinergic drugs are favored in demented individuals because of the relationship between cognitive function and acetylcholine. Selective serotonin reuptake inhibitors (SSRIs) should be avoided in treating agitated patients as they can cause worsening of the agitation.

Other Drug Choices

β-Adrenergic blockers, particularly the noncardioselective type, such as propranolol (Inderal), have been used to treat agitation and aggressive behavior in some demented patients. Carbamazepine (Tegretol) is being tested in clinical trials to decrease hostility and agitation.

Overall Approach to the Patient with Dementia

The overall care of a patient with dementia requires close attention to the following guidelines:

1. Avoid medications—Virtually all medications can cause and/or worsen cognitive disabilities and a decline in functional status. An effort should be made to prescribe as few drugs as possible.
2. Provide behavioral counseling—Demented patients and their families will benefit from counseling regarding the following issues:
   • The disease and its progression and prognosis
   • Anticipated behavioral changes
   • Community resources for long-term care needs and family-support groups
   • Advance directives/durable powers of attorney for health care
3. Provide cognitive support—Counsel families about the ways in which they can help patients with dementia continue to function at their peak intellectual level:
   • Maintain consistency in the daily routine; avoid changes in the environment.
   • Provide sufficient lighting during evening hours.
   • Provide daily reminders for orientation: calendars, pictures, clocks, newspapers.
   • Develop mechanisms to use intact intellect—games, puzzles, activities.
   • Allow and support reminiscing about the past.
   • Avoid usurping tasks or conversations and avoid overcorrecting or criticizing.
   • Foster continued socialization.

PATIENT AND FAMILY EDUCATION
Caregivers

Caregivers of patients with dementia require ongoing education and support. The vast majority of care is provided by relatives. The burden experienced in providing care is the primary factor determining how long the patient remains in the home. Ever-increasing needs of the patient will overwhelm the unprepared caregiver. Support for caregivers includes addressing psychologic, social, financial, and legal issues; many community-based resources are available to provide such support. Anticipatory guidance for the many problems that caregivers face is crucial. The availability and use of respite services such as day care or parent-sitting services can be very helpful.

Education

The management of dementia involves providing patients and their families with sufficient education and resources to assist in this devastating illness. The two most useful resources are the Alzheimer's Disease Association, which has national and local chapters (national office: 800-272-3900), and the classic text, *The 36 Hour Day,* by Mace and Rabins, published by Johns

Hopkins University Press (available for $12 from the publisher at 800-537-5487).

FOLLOW-UP

Follow-up visits for the patient with dementia should be scheduled every 3 to 6 months, or more frequently if needed, and should address the following issues:

- Treatment of comorbid conditions
- Evaluation of ongoing medications
- Evaluation for behavioral disturbances
- For family and caregivers, assessment of social and legal issues, and encouragement to use respite services and psychologic support services
- Establishment of programs to maintain behavior such as daily exercise and socialization activities
- Encouragement of caregivers to modulate environment by reducing stimulation, providing clocks and various media to reinforce time/date orientation, and ensuring safety by reducing hot-water temperature and by fireproofing living quarters
- Promotion of safety by advising patient to stop driving and to wear name tags and medic-alert identification.

SUGGESTED READINGS

Costa P Jr, Williams T, et al. Recognition and initial assessment of Alzheimer's disease and related dementias: clinical practice guidelines. Agency for Health Care Policy and Research Publication No. 97-0702, 1996.

Gauthier S, ed. Clinical diagnosis and management of Alzheimer's disease. Boston: Butterworth-Heinemann, 1996.

Geldmacher D, Whitehouse P. Evaluation of dementia. N Engl J Med 1996;335: 330–336.

Helms P. Efficacy of antipsychotics in the treatment of the behavioral complications of dementia: a review of the literature. J Am Geriatr Soc 1985;33:206–209.

Small GW, et al. Diagnosis and treatment of Alzheimer disease and related disorders. JAMA 1997;278:1363–1371.

Tangalos E. The mini-mental state examination in general medical practice: clinical utility and acceptance. Mayo Clin Proc 1996;71:829–837.

Winograd C, Jarvik L. Physician management of the demented patient. J Am Geriatr Soc 1986;34:295–309.

CHAPTER 4

Depression in the Elderly

Depression that begins early in life and recurrent episodes that occur in later life may be different from depression that has its onset late in life. Depression with a late-life onset is more commonly associated with underlying brain abnormalities; some are not diagnosed until years after the first presentation of depression. Brain imaging in these patients shows enlargement of the ventricles and increased intensity of the white matter. There is a higher incidence of subsequent dementia among such patients and a more chronic course of the depressive symptoms. Major depression, with all of the classic vegetative and cognitive symptoms, does occur in the elderly; however, more elders have dysthymia or even a lesser illness referred to as subsyndromal depression. Depression in the elderly is a spectrum disorder rather than a clear-category disease state. Also, differentiating clinically significant depression from minor mood fluctuations or from underlying physical illnesses is a challenge. Although routine screening for depression in asymptomatic individuals of all ages is not recommended, clinicians need to have a high index of suspicion in older adults, who are at higher risk for depression. The American College of Physicians recommends that older adults undergo screening of their emotional status.

TYPES OF DEPRESSION

Major Depression

Major depression is defined as depressed mood or a marked loss of interest that is experienced most of the day, nearly every day, for 2 weeks or longer. In addition, at least five of the following eight symptoms must be present during the same 2-week period, representing a change from previous functioning:

- Unexplained weight loss or weight gain of more than 5% in 1 month, or loss of appetite
- Insomnia or hypersomnia
- Psychomotor agitation or retardation
- Fatigue or loss of energy

- Feelings of worthlessness or guilt
- Diminished concentration
- Thoughts of death; suicidal ideation
- Loss of interest or pleasure in daily activities

Dysthymia

Dysthymia is defined as a chronic depression with mild to moderate symptoms that lasts 2 years or longer, occurring on most days. Dysthymia does not fulfill all of the criteria for major depression. Diagnosis can be made when a minimum of two of the above symptoms are detected. Brief periods of normal mood can occur. Major depression and dysthymia can coexist as double depression. This is more difficult to treat than major depression. Personality disorders and chronic medical conditions can also coexist with dysthymia.

Subsyndromal Depression

Subsyndromal depression is defined as levels of depressive symptoms associated with increased risk of major depression, physical disabilities, medical illness, and/or a high use of health-care services. Symptoms do not meet criteria for major depression or dysthymia, but are significant enough to cause morbidity and compromised quality of life.

CHIEF COMPLAINT

The presenting complaint in patients with depression is frequently nonspecific and atypical and commonly looks like a variety of physical illnesses. Sadness is frequently a presenting sign of depression, although not every patient has this complaint. Common complaints are listed in Table 4.1.

HISTORY

The database is crucial to the diagnosis of depression. Because of the association of depression with a variety of medical illnesses, medications, and nondisease issues, each elderly patient with suspected depression must be evaluated for an underlying medical condition. Likewise, individuals with diagnosed medical conditions should be considered at risk for a concomitant depression.

Risk factors for depression include the following:

- Medications
- Concurrent medical disorder
- Life stressors (recent) and lack of social supports
- Prior episode of depression
- Family history of major depressive disorder
- Personal history of suicide attempt
- Substance abuse

TABLE 4.1. Somatised Symptoms of Depression

System	Symptoms
General	Fatigue
	Weight loss
	Anorexia
	Anxiety
	Insomnia
	Weakness
	Paranoia
	Apathy
Cardiac	Chest pains
	Palpitations
	Fainting
Pulmonary	Shortness of breath
Gastrointestinal	Nausea
	Abdominal pain
	Diarrhea/constipation
Genitourinary	Dysuria
	Frequency of urination
	Urgency
	Incontinence
	Sexual function problems (e.g., impotence, dyspareunia)
Musculoskeletal	Diffuse myalgias/arthralgias
	Back pain
Neurologic	Memory difficulty
	Concentration loss
	Parasthesias
	Headache
	Dizziness

The classic symptoms of depression can be easily remembered with the mnemonic SIGE CAPS, which can be used in screening history:

- Sleep disturbance
- Interest, lack of

EPIDEMIOLOGIC CONSIDERATIONS

Among community-dwelling elders, major depression occurs in less than 1%, dysthymia in 2%, and subsyndromal depression in 13 to 27%. Among hospitalized elders, major depression can be found in 10% and dysthymia and subsyndromal depression in up to 30%. Among nursing home elders, major depression has a prevalence of 12%, whereas dysthymia and subsyndromal depression have a prevalence of close to 50%. Depression occurs more commonly in women than in men in the young, and this remains the same for the elderly age group. However, depression in the elderly does have some significant differences from the disease in younger patients: Apathy, withdrawal, and cognitive impairment are seen more commonly in the elderly. Older adult men have the single highest suicide rate of any age group. Psychotic (delusional) depression is more common in the elderly than in the young.

- Guilt
- Energy loss
- Concentration difficulty
- Appetite alteration
- Psychomotor retardation or agitation
- Suicidal ideation

Given the prevalence of depression and the difficulty in diagnosing it, depression screening is considered a part of formal geriatric assessment. Some screening method should be a routine component of office evaluations. The commonly used forms or tools for such screening are the Beck Depression Inventory and the Zung Depression Scale. The standard use of these forms has been recommended; however, their length makes them cumbersome for practical office screening. A faster way of screening for the family physician is to ask every patient questions about the following:

- Sad or depressed mood
- Social withdrawal
- Sleep disturbances (persistent sleep problems are commonly associated with depression in the elderly)

An important component of history-taking for depression in the elderly involves the issue of suicide. Suicide rates are the highest of all age groups in elderly men. A majority of depressed suicide victims have seen a primary care physician in the last month prior to their suicide, with close to 40% seeing the physician in the last week. Certainly, elderly patients who have depressive symptoms should be asked directly about suicidal thoughts or plans. Suicide ranks among the top 10 causes of death in the elderly. Major risk factors for suicide, in addition to depression, include the following:

- Male gender
- Caucasian race
- Widowed, divorced, or separated
- Low economic status
- Poor health status
- Alcohol abuse

Other factors suggesting suicide risk include recent deaths that induce loneliness, financial problems, or a change in health status. Elderly suicide victims most often use guns or hang themselves, whereas those who attempt suicide, but fail, often overdose on drugs. Suicide is one of the most important preventable causes of death in the elderly.

Depression occurs as a side effect of many of the medications used to treat the common chronic diseases in the elderly (Table 4.2). The complex interplay of depression, physical illness, and medications is important for the family physician to recognize and carefully manage.

Surprisingly, cancer is associated with depression much less often than ex-

TABLE 4.2. Medications Known to Cause Depression

Methyldopa (Aldomet)
Barbiturates
Benzodiazepines
Chlorpromazine (Thorazine)
Cimetidine (Tagamet)
Clonidine (Catapres)
Corticosteroids
Digitalis
Estrogens
Guanethidine (Ismelin)
Haloperidol (Haldol)
Hydralazine (Apresoline)
Indomethacin (Indocin)
Levodopa (Larodopa)
Opioid analgesics
Progesterone
Propoxyphene (Darvon)
Propranolol (Inderal)
Psychostimulants
Reserpine (Serpasil)
Tamoxifen (Nolvadex)
Vinblastine (Velban)
Vincristine (Oncovin)

TABLE 4.3. Non–Disease-Specific Issues of Depression and Illness in the Elderly

Situation	Comments
Acute illness	Abrupt loss of function, disability, and fear of death
Chronic disease	Progressive loss and dependency, lack of control, inevitability
Hospitalization	Loss of control, isolation, deprivation, infantilization, immobilization
Damage to body image	Amputation, cancer with surgical loss (e.g., breast, prostate), acute myocardial infarction
Loss	Death of spouse, family, and friends
Pain	Chronicity, severity, anticipatory

pected. Non–disease-specific issues also can cause depression and illness in the elderly. Examples are given in Table 4.3.

There is a higher incidence of major depression and subsyndromal impairment in patients who have experienced a loss. The boundary between pathology and nonpathology is indistinct and based primarily on severity of the symptoms. It is inappropriate to base the decision to treat on any specified time frame, as many people can continue to have symptoms for years after the death of a loved one. Major depression is estimated to occur in up to 15% of bereaved persons in up to 2 to 3 years following a loss. The family physician should continue to question patients who have experienced a significant loss.

PHYSICAL EXAMINATION

The physical exam has a limited role in the evaluation of depressed patients. The primary focus is differentiating physical diseases from the changes associated with the affective disorder. Differentiating weight loss from the anorexia of depression versus that from an occult malignancy is often a challenge. A careful look is necessary for the physical findings of thyroid or neurologic disease. Other organ-system pathologies that occur in the elderly should also be evaluated as potential contributors to depression (see Table 4.4).

Mental-Status Exam

Depression can be etiologic in creating cognitive dysfunction. Some depressed patients will have as their major manifestation a significant cognitive loss, which can be misdiagnosed as a dementia. This pseudodementia is sometimes difficult to diagnose. These patients will typically answer questions with "I don't know" or "I don't care." A trial of antidepressants may be the way this illness is recognized.

DIAGNOSTIC TESTS

Routine diagnostic testing of older patients with depression is often done to rule out organic illnesses and to provide baseline information prior to initiation of medication therapy.

Standard blood tests include complete blood count (CBC), B_{12} levels, thyroid function tests, syphilis serology, and serum electrolytes. A computed tomographic (CT) scan is indicated if there is suspicion of a detectable organic disorder based on history or physical findings. The clinical yield without such suspicion is low. An electrocardiogram and measures of serum creatinine and blood urea nitrogen (BUN) will be helpful in planning therapy.

TABLE 4.4. Medical Conditions Associated With or Causing Depression

Condition	Factors Leading to or Associated With Depression
Malignancies	
Any site	Pain, disability, and dependency
Pancreas	Anorexia, weight loss, back pain, and depression are common presentations
CNS—frontal lobes	Apathy and depression; abnormal behavior
Neurologic	
Stroke	Frustration, disability, and dependency
Subdural hematomas	Decreased awareness, cognitive loss, depression
Neurodegenerative diseases [amyotrophic lateral sclerosis (ALS), multiple sclerosis (MS), Alzheimer's, Parkinson's]	Cognitive loss, dependency
Thyroid	
Hypothyroidism	Psychomotor retardation, slowed reflexes, depressed effect
Hyperthyroidism	Apathetic hyperthyroidism with psychomotor retardation and depression
Hyperparathyroidism	Hypercalcemia, apathy, fatigue, bone pain, and depression
Rheumatologic illness	Chronic pain, disability, dependency, steroid use
Cardiopulmonary	
Congestive heart failure (CHF)	Dyspnea, dependency
Myocardial infarction (MI)	Disability, fear, dependency, and depression
Chronic obstructive pulmonary disease (COPD)	Dependency, fear, anxiety, dyspnea
Genitourinary	
Renal failure	Uremic symptoms of fatigue, nausea, impending dialysis

DIFFERENTIAL DIAGNOSIS

The following should be considered in the differential diagnosis of depression in an elderly patient:

Bipolar illness is rare in the elderly. Manic episodes can be typical, with elevated mood, grandiosity, hyperactivity, and flight of ideas, or they can present as cognitive dysfunction, disorientation, and delirium. Patients with late-life-onset mania, like those with depression occurring in old age, typically have an underlying brain disorder (e.g., tumor, stroke).

Depression can be mixed with other psychiatric illnesses such as borderline personality disorder, schizophrenia, or other delusional disorders. A common association in the elderly is depression and a generalized anxiety disorder. Anxiety syndromes are common in elders with medical illnesses, and depression is a common denominator in many cases.

Medications listed in Table 4.2 may be responsible for depression. Alcoholism and depression are linked in the elderly as in the young. It is estimated that alcohol abuse occurs in up to 10% of the current elderly population. Alcohol is a depressant, and chronic alcohol use can produce symptoms of classic depression. Similarly, alcohol consumption is used by many in an attempt to alleviate the psychologic pain of depression.

Bereavement and grief are not diseases, but are often confused with depression in the elderly. It is commonplace to experience a loss of a loved one, family, or friend. Although this loss can be the trigger of a depressive episode, most individuals experience a mild, nondisease set of symptoms referred to as bereavement and grief. The symptoms include both affective and somatic complaints similar to depression. Common symptoms include a preoccupation with the memory of the dying person, even so far as hearing their voice or seeing their image, and a feeling of intense sadness with frequent crying spells. Symptoms of bereavement are commonly more intense around key dates such as anniversaries, birthdays, holidays, or the date of the death. These are normal features of a nonpathologic grieving.

WHEN TO REFER

The family physician is and must be the lead health-care resource for the depressed elderly. Referral is indicated if treatment is ineffective or there is

TABLE 4.5. Reasons for Referral of Older Adults with Depression

Patient is suicidal
Patient has severe psychotic depression
Hospitalization is considered because of psychotic symptoms
Complex disease with multiple symptoms
To obtain a second opinion

question about the diagnosis. Other potential reasons for referral are listed in Table 4.5. In many communities there are psychiatrists or psychologists who specialize in the care of the depressed elderly. Formal psychotherapy will most likely be a referral for most family physicians, although the techniques are not restricted to any specific medical discipline.

MANAGEMENT

General Issues

The goals of therapy are initially to relieve symptoms and to prevent relapses and recurrences while always focusing on the patient's functional abilities and quality of life. The three phases of treatment include the following:

- Six to 12 weeks of treatment to relieve symptoms
- Ongoing treatment for up to 9 months to prevent relapse
- Maintenance treatment when necessary

The main treatment options for depressive symptoms include the following:

- Psychologic counseling
- Antidepressant medications
- Electroconvulsive therapy (ECT)
- A combination of any or all of the above

Psychologic support should be offered and encouraged in all patients irrespective of the chosen treatment methods.

Formal Psychologic Counseling

Psychologic support should be offered and fostered for all bereaved individuals. An empathetic ear can comfort all who grieve. Formal support services through counseling, group therapy, or individual psychotherapy can benefit some grieving patients. Formal psychotherapy is particularly beneficial in the elderly who cannot or will not take antidepressant medications or who are dealing with clear interpersonal stressors. In most situations this will require a referral to a skilled therapist. Although no standard techniques have shown consistent advantages, two modalities of formal psychologic counseling have been demonstrated in formal research to be efficacious in treating the elderly: cognitive-behavioral therapy and interpersonal therapy.

Cognitive-behavioral therapy is designed to train patients to identify and correct negative thoughts that are key to the depressive symptoms. This approach is based on learning theories linking cognitive function with behavioral outcomes. Cognitive restructuring helps the depressed elder to avoid overgeneralizations and catastrophic negative thinking and to think in terms of reality. Behavioral components of this approach involve focusing on positive life experiences and pleasurable activities.

Interpersonal therapy is based on the relationships that surround a depressed individual's life. Focusing on the individual's roles, role transitions, role disputes, and self image are the backbone of this therapy. Interpersonal therapy fosters the enhancement of positive and the avoidance of negative relationships.

Key to both cognitive-behavioral and interpersonal therapy is a relatively cognitively intact person. Patients with moderate dementias will not benefit from formal psychotherapy. Families and caregivers of all elderly patients, even demented individuals, can and should be involved in formal psychotherapeutic interventions. Not only can this involvement benefit the patient, but depressive symptoms are more common in these individuals as well.

Pharmacotherapy

Medications to treat depression are highly efficacious and safe. Antidepressants should always be used when depressive symptoms negatively affect a person's quality of life or functional status. Additional indications for medication treatment are given in Table 4.6. It is not necessary to have a diagnosis of major depression or to wait for severe symptoms to initiate drug therapy. Even patients with subsyndromal depression, in which a patient with mild symptoms has not responded quickly to informal or formal counseling, can benefit from antidepressant medications. The family physician should be facile with the use of the major antidepressant medications (Table 4.7). General recommendations for the use of antidepressants are to achieve adequate dosages for a sufficient length of time. Older adults should be started with low dosages of medication. Drug interactions also are common in older adults, and concurrent medication review is essential. It is common for antidepressants to take a minimum of 2 weeks and usually 6 to 8 weeks before a therapeutic response is noted. An adequate trial is considered a minimum of 8 weeks before labeling a particular drug as ineffective.

The length of therapy in the elderly should be longer, given the higher risk of relapse in this age group. All patients should be given ongoing therapy for

TABLE 4.6.   Indications for Pharmacotherapy for Depression in the Elderly

Severe symptoms
Recurrences
Psychotic features
Melancholia
Prior response to medication
Combination with psychotherapy

TABLE 4.7.   Antidepressant Medications Commonly Used in the Elderly

Medication Class	Commonly Used Drugs	Dosages	Advantages	Disadvantages
Tricyclic and heterocyclic antidepressants (TCAs)[a]	Nortriptyline (Pamelor) Desipramine (Norpramin)	Nortriptyline: 1 mg per kg Desipramine: 1.5 to 2 mg per kg Smaller doses may be effective in relieving some symptoms, such as insomnia or low mood. Target blood levels are 50 to 150 ng per mL for nortriptyline and above 125 ng per mL for desipramine.	Well researched and established efficacy.	Sedative; encourages weight gain Anticholinergic side effects: prostatic obstruction, cognitive dysfunction, cardiac arrhythmias
	Trazadone (Desyrel)	Trazodone: 50 to 300 mg per day. Blood levels are not available.	Sedative; lack of anticholinergic side effects	Orthostasis, priapism, drowsiness
Selective serotonin reuptake inhibitors (SSRIs)[a]	Fluoxetine (Prozac) Paroxetine (Paxil) Sertraline (Zoloft)	Fluoxetine and paroxetine: 10 to 20 mg per day Sertraline: 50 to 100 mg per day Blood levels are not available.	Lack of anticholinergic side effects	Nausea, diarrhea, insomnia, agitation, anxiety, SIADH (syndrome of inappropriate antidiuretic hormone), drug interactions, anorgasmia, extrapyramidal movements, serotonin syndrome of restlessness, mental status changes, fever
Monamine oxidase Inhibitors (MAOI)	Tranylcypromine (Parnate) Phenelzine (Nardil)	Tranylcypromine: 20 to 30 mg per day Phenelzine: 15 to 45 mg per day	Efficacy in nonresponders to TCAs or SSRIs; effective against panic attacks	Hypertension with food and drug interactions; orthostatic hypotension

continued

TABLE 4.7. *continued*

Medication Class	Most Commonly Used Drugs	Dosages	Advantages	Disadvantages
Others	Bupropion (Wellbutrin) Venlafaxine (Effexor) Nefazodone (Serzone)	Bupropion: 75 to 100 mg per day Venlafaxine: 75 mg per day in two to three divided doses Nefazadone: 100 mg per day	No cardiac toxicity; useful when others fail	Hypertension, seizures, SSRI-like side effects
	Methylphenidate (Ritalin)[b]	5 to 15 mg three times per day	Rapid onset, effective for hospitalized elders needing rehabilitation	Short-term use only; agitation

[a]In SSRI/TCA combination therapy, the dosages of the TCAs should be reduced, as they are metabolized via the hepatic p450 system. The combination decreases the anxiety and insomnia related to SSRIs. The SSRI is typically prescribed as a daytime dose, with the TCA given at night to take advantage of its sedative effects. The reduced TCA dosage lessens the anticholinergic side effects of the combination.

[b]Not currently approved by the U.S. Food and Drug Administration for the treatment of depression in the elderly.

at least 6 months, if not 1 year, after symptoms have resolved. In many patients maintenance therapy may be considered indefinitely.

Tricyclic Antidepressants (TCAs)

TCAs are the best-studied medications for the treatment of depression in the elderly. Nortriptyline (Pamelor) and desipramine (Norpramin) have lower anticholinergic side effects and less sedation than amitryptiline (Elavil) or imipramine (Tofranil) and are therefore preferred for use in the elderly.

Side Effects. TCAs have fallen out of favor recently because of their side effects. Many patients experience transient dry mouth, mild constipation, urinary hesitation, and orthostatic hypotension. Serious cardiac side effects have raised concern over the use of TCAs in many elderly patients. TCAs have been implicated in inducing life-threatening arrhythmias in patients with preexisting cardiac disease and in aggravating heart block. TCAs should be avoided in patients with urinary obstruction from prostatic disease and preexisting cognitive dysfunction because they will worsen the symptoms of these diseases.

An important issue is the toxicity of overdoses with TCAs. These drugs produce significant cardiac conduction disease when taken in large doses. It is best to avoid prescribing TCAs to potentially suicidal patients. If it is necessary, only a small number of pills should be dispensed at a time; commonly less than 1 g is recommended.

Trazadone

Trazadone (Desyrel) is a heterocyclic similar to the TCAs; however, it has low anticholinergic properties but high sedative properties. It is a good choice in elders who require sedation but who cannot tolerate anticholinergic side effects. An elderly patient with an agitated depression who has a dementing illness may be an ideal candidate for trazadone.

Side Effects.   A unique, although rare, side effect of trazadone is priapism.

Selective Serotonin Reuptake Inhibitors (SSRIs)

Clinical trials have demonstrated that SSRIs are as effective as TCAs in treating mild to moderate depression in the elderly. However, TCAs are more effective than SSRIs in the treatment of severe depression. The side effects related to SSRIs are less pronounced than those of TCAs, making the SSRIs a common first choice in deciding therapy. The three current SSRIs available for treating depression are fluoxetine (Prozac), paroxetine (Paxil), and sertraline (Zoloft), and these are roughly equivalent in efficacy and side effects.

Side Effects.   The common side effects of SSRIs are nausea, diarrhea, headache, insomnia, anxiety, and agitation. SSRIs also can induce an extrapyramidal movement disorder that mimics Parkinson's disease and can cause Syndrome of Inappropriate Antidiuretic Hormone (SIADH). Fluoxetine has been associated with orgasmic dysfunction in women. SSRIs also block the hepatic cytochrome p450 system, and drugs that are metabolized by this system will accumulate in the body. Overdoses of SSRIs are relatively benign, especially when compared with the toxicity seen with TCA overdoses.

Combination Therapy with TCAs and SSRIs

The combined use of TCAs and SSRIs is generally safe and effective in treating some depressed elderly patients. A common use is a full-dose SSRI taken in the morning with a low dose of a sedating TCA at bedtime. This is useful in patients who experience insomnia with SSRIs, as well as in those who are receiving SSRIs because of the potential side effects of the TCAs but who have insomnia as a major feature of depression. Other combinations such as an antidepressant and a benzodiazepine anxiolytic may be useful in some cases.

Monoamine Oxidase Inhibitors (MAO) Inhibitors

MAO inhibitors are used infrequently to treat depression in the elderly. They are effective and have few cardiac side effects. The two available medications are phenelzine (Nardil) and tranylcypromine (Parnate). Use of MAOI may be considered in patients with panic attacks and depression or in patients with heart blocks and arrhythmias.

Side Effects. MAO inhibitors cause orthostatic hypotension and have interactions with the following foods and drugs that produce severe hypertensive reactions:

- Beer
- Beans
- Figs (canned)
- Cheeses
- Chicken liver
- Chocolate
- Red wine
- Processed meats
- Sympathomimetics (over-the-counter decongestants)
- Demerol
- Methyldopa (Aldomet)
- Levodopa (Laradopa)

Other Medications

There are a group of old and new drugs that have a role in the treatment of depression in the elderly. Bupropion (Wellbutrin) is a new stimulating antidepressant that can be used in elders whose depressive symptoms include psychomotor retardation, fatigue, and poor motivation. It has no cardiac toxicity and can be used in patients with known heart disease. Daily doses are usually 75 to 100 mg three to four times a day. Side effects include tremor, hypertension, and seizures. Patients with a history of seizures should avoid using bupropion.

Venlafaxine (Effexor) and nefazodone (Serzone) are new medications that inhibit serotonin and norepinephrine uptake. Both of these drugs are useful if other drugs fail. They have similar side effects to SSRIs, have little anticholinergic actions, and have no cardiac toxicity.

Methylphenidate (Ritalin) is a stimulant that has been used for years for a variety of illnesses and is in common use today for the treatment of attention-deficit and hyperactivity disorders (ADHD) in children. It is not currently approved by the U.S. Food and Drug Administration for the treatment of depression in the elderly, although it can be an excellent drug for the treatment of depression in medically ill elders who are apathetic and lack motivation. Methylphenidate has a rapid onset of action, and results can be seen within days of drug initiation. It has been used successfully in elderly hospital patients whose depressive apathy prevents them from participating in rehabilitation programs. The drug should be limited to less than 1 month of therapy, and side effects are rare. If effective, a TCA or SSRI should be initiated for longer term therapy.

Methylphenidate is contraindicated in patients with severe hypertension or unstable angina.

Electroconvulsive Therapy (ECT)

ECT is the most effective treatment for severe, persistent, or refractory depression. It is particularly effective for depressed patients with psychotic features or strong suicidal ideation. It is a much maligned modality that should be used far more than it is currently. ECT provides a rapid relief of symptoms and has a minimum of side effects. Treatments are usually given three times a week for a total of six to twelve times. The success rate, in patients in whom drug therapy has failed, is up to 80%.

Side Effects

Common side effects of ECT include confusion and a short-duration memory impairment. Spacing the ECT treatments to once or twice a week can reduce these cognitive changes, but will delay the reduction of depressive symptoms. The most serious complications are cardiac, including myocardial infarctions, arrhythmias, and worsening congestive heart failure, which can occur within a few hours of ECT. Patients with known cardiac disease should be closely monitored, adequately hydrated and oxygenated, and given prophylactic β-blockers prior to their treatments. Overall the mortality rate with ECT is 0.01%. ECT is effective and safe in patients with known dementia disorders; however, the cognitive changes related to ECT can persist longer than in cognitively intact patients. ECT is contraindicated in patients with intracranial tumors, hydrocephalus, and within 1 month of an acute cerebrovascular accident.

Additional Management Considerations

When symptoms become severe, interrupting the individual's ability to function, or when specific symptoms are a major feature (such as persistent loss of appetite, insomnia, or suicidal behavior), antidepressant medication should be initiated. If ECT is the chosen modality for attaining relief from symptoms, if medication and counseling have proved ineffective, antidepressant medications should be administered on completion as maintenance treatment. ECT is a useful modality in the elderly despite its lack of commonplace availability. Referral for ECT may be appropriate in some cases. Informal psychologic support is the backbone to any therapy, and this can be obtained through a variety of resources. Assisting the depressed elder in utilizing these resources is an important role of the family physician. Informal empathetic support from family, friends, social organizations, or churches can be the key to getting back to a normal lifestyle for many elders. In fact, encouraging socialization is important in preventing depression in the elderly.

FOLLOW-UP

The association of depression with physical illnesses and medications is a significant issue. Depression coexisting with, or as a component of, an underlying chronic illness occurs regularly in the elderly. In these situations it is clear that morbidity, mortality, and functional loss are more significant than in patients who have the same level of chronic disease without depression. Depression is a disease that is characterized by relapses and recurrent episodes. Depressed patients use medical services excessively, with an increase in physician visits, medication use, emergency room visits, and hospitalizations. In fact, a single depressive episode increases an elder's risk for subsequent declines in health and functional status. Patients diagnosed with depression should be followed closely to optimize their therapy and reduce their risks of subsequent diseases. The medications used to treat depression have significant side effects that need close monitoring. All patients receiving TCAs should undergo periodic electrocardiograms to evaluate for heart block. A prolongation of any intervals, PR, QRS, QT, should cause the physician to reevaluate continued use of TCAs and/or to reduce the dosages. Effective drug therapy should be continued for a minimum of 6 months to 1 year. Patients should be followed for relapses and recurrent episodes. Some patients will require continued drug therapy for the duration of their lives.

PATIENT EDUCATION

The following are key points to convey to patients:

- It usually takes 10 days to 3 weeks of medication before improvements occur.
- The sedative effects of the medication will help insomnia, and improved sleep will enhance outlook.
- Medications are usually taken for 6 months and then a drug holiday may be considered. However, medication may be necessary indefinitely.
- Socialization is important. Increased involvement in social activities (such as visiting child-care centers, church, bingo, and meals with groups) often improves outlook.
- Exercise is also helpful in improving mood. Patients should increase the activities they find pleasurable.
- Support groups are helpful.

Resources to recommend to patients include the following:

- *Depression is a Treatable Illness: A Patients Guide.* Agency For Health Care Policy And Research Publications Clearinghouse, PO Box 8547, Silver Spring, MD 20907 (telephone: 800-358-9295).
- *Depression: What You Need to Know; If You're Over 65 and Feeling Depressed; Helping the Depressed Person Get Treatment; What to Do When a Friend Is Depressed; La Depresion Existen Tratamientos Ecaces;* and many other materials. DEPRESSION Awareness, Recognition, and Treat-

ment (D/ART) Public Education Campaign, 5600 Fishers Lane, Rm 14C-02,* Rockville, MD 20857 (telephone 800-421-4211).

Suggested readings

Hoenig HG, George LK, Meador KG, et al. Use of antidepressants by non-psychiatrists in the treatment of medically ill depressed elderly. Am J Psychiatr 1997;154:1369-1375.

Lebowtiz BD, Pearson JL, Schneider LS, et al. Diagnosis and treatment of depression in late life—consensus statement update. JAMA 1997;278:1186-1190.

NIH Consensus Conference. Diagnosis and treatment of depression in late life. JAMA 1992;268:1018-1024.

Rigler SK, Studenski S, Duncan PN, xet al. Pharmacologic treatment of geriatric depression: key issues in interpreting the evidence. J Am Geriatr Soc 1998;46:106-110.

CHAPTER 5
....

Hypertension

High blood pressure in the elderly is not benign and is not a normal consequence of aging. Hypertension has been proved conclusively to be a risk factor for cardiovascular and cerebrovascular morbidity and mortality. In elderly patients treatment of both systolic and diastolic hypertension has been shown to reduce these risks. Therefore diagnosing and treating hypertension should be a primary goal in the care of the elderly.

Hypertension in the elderly is a distinctly different disease than in the young. In the young hypertension is associated with alterations in the renin-angiotensin system, obesity, and insulin and renal dysfunction. In the elderly hypertension is more commonly a result of vascular-resistance alterations in all vessels from the aorta to the smallest arterioles. These alterations result from atherosclerotic changes, loss of compliance in vessel walls, and changes in the β-adrenergic and α-adrenergic tone.

Recent studies have demonstrated that an elevated pulse pressure (systolic blood pressure minus diastolic blood pressure), indicating reduced vascular compliance in large arteries, may more accurately assess cardiovascular risk than either number in the blood pressure alone.

CHIEF COMPLAINT

Patients with hypertension are generally asymptomatic, although they commonly attribute many nonspecific symptoms to elevated blood pressure (headache, dizziness, anxiety). True symptoms develop when hypertension is very severe or causes end-organ damage. Common, true hypertensive symptoms in the elderly are the result of the following: (1) macrovascular disease—damage to the brain with dementia or stroke and damage to the heart with angina and heart failure; and (2) microvascular disease—damage to the kidney with renal insufficiency and failure and damage to the eye with retinal vascular disease.

HISTORY

The purpose of the history and physical exam is to (1) search for a specific cause of hypertension, (2) identify concomitant diseases, (3) document end-

EPIDEMIOLOGIC CONSIDERATIONS

The prevalence of hypertension in the elderly is influenced by the effect of age on blood pressure:
- Systolic pressure increases linearly with age, up to age 75, with the rate of increase being steeper for women than men.
- Diastolic pressure similarly increases with age; however, it plateaus by about age 60.
- Isolated systolic hypertension affects approximately 10% of patients at age 70 and 20% of patients at age 80.
- Combined systolic/diastolic hypertension occurs in close to 50% of patients over age 65.

organ damage, and (4) determine patients functional capacity. When taking the history, it is important to seek information on the following:

History of present illness
- Duration and management of any prior hypertension

Previous vascular disease
- Coronary heart disease
- Heart failure
- Cerebrovascular disease
- Peripheral vascular disease
- Renal disease
- Retinal disease

Other risk factors for vascular disease progression
- Diabetes mellitus
- Smoking history
- Dyslipidemia
- Family history of vascular disease
- Other comorbid conditions
- Gout
- Sexual dysfunction
- Hyperthyroidism

History to determine etiology
- Recent weight change
- Decreased physical activity
- Diet, concentrating on salt intake
- Medications, including herbal remedies, over-the-counter preparations, illicit drugs

Psychologic and environmental factors that may affect blood pressure control
- Employment status
- Psychosocial history
- Working conditions
- Activities of daily living
- Cognitive function

PHYSICAL EXAMINATION

The critical first step in diagnosing and managing older adults with hypertension is accurate blood pressure measurements (Table 5.1). Most family physicians use the office blood pressure cuff as their diagnostic tool. There are a number of important points to consider in determining office blood pressures in the elderly:

- Proper cuff size
- Measurements in both arms
- Measurements should be taken with the patient sitting with back supported and after at least 5 minutes of rest and standing after 1 to 2 minutes
- At least two measurements, at least 2 minutes apart, should be taken at each of three visits

Ambulatory blood pressure monitoring appears to correlate more closely than clinical blood pressure with a variety of measures of target–organ damage such as left ventricular hypertrophy. This procedure is most helpful in patients with suspected "white coat" hypertension, but may be helpful also in patients with episodic hypertension or hypotension. It is not recommended for routine blood pressure screening.

TABLE 5.1. Classification of Blood Pressure in Adults[a]

	Systolic (mm Hg)	Diastolic (mm Hg)
Optimal	< 120 and	< 80
Normal	< 130 and	< 85
High normal	130 to 139 or	85 to 90
Mild (stage 1) hypertension	140–159 or	90 to 99
Moderate (stage 2) hypertension	160–179 or	100 to 109
Severe (stage 3) hypertension	≥ 180 or	≥ 110
Isolated systolic hypertension	> 160 and	< 90

[a]Based on two or more readings taken at each of 2 or more visits after the initial screening.

Adapted from The sixth report of the Joint National Committee on Prevention, Detection, Evaluation, and Treatment of High Blood Pressure. Arch Intern Med 1997;157:2413–2446.

The remainder of the evaluation includes the following:

- Vital signs, including height, weight, waist circumference
- Fundoscopic exam for hypertensive retinopathy
- Neck exam for carotid bruits or enlarged thyroid
- Cardiac exam for rate or rhythm abnormality, precordial heave, murmurs, third or fourth heart sounds
- Lung exam for rales, bronchospasm
- Abdominal exam for bruits, enlarged kidneys, masses, abnormal aortic pulsations
- Extremities for diminished peripheral arterial pulses, edema
- Neurologic assessment, including auscultation, coordination, manual dexterity, and mental status
- Functional capacity evaluation is critical in determining patient's ability to perform activities of daily living and to manage care of hypertension

DIAGNOSTIC TESTS

All hypertensive patients should undergo baseline laboratory testing to look for intrinsic renal disease, unrecognized diabetes, hyperlipidemia, and end-organ status (Table 5.2). These tests may be repeated on an annual basis to follow the status of the end organs affected by hypertension.

Captopril renography is the currently preferred noninvasive test if renovascular hypertension is suspected. This test is based on the principle that suppression of the renin-angiotensin system in the presence of a hemodynamically significant renal artery stenosis will result in a decrease in the glomerular filtration rate in the affected kidney. It utilizes nuclear scanning technology and has 91% sensitivity and 94% specificity. It does require that the patient stop taking antihypertensive agents for an adequate length of time prior to the study. Arteriography is the gold standard for diagnosing renal artery stenosis. Suspicion of the possibility of renal artery stenosis occurs in the setting of the following:

- Hypertension
- Poor response to treatment
- Increased blood pressure after a period of good control
- Sudden onset of increased blood pressure

DIFFERENTIAL DIAGNOSIS

Once the diagnosis of hypertension has been established, an effort should be made to diagnose identifiable causes (Table 5.3). In most cases hypertension will be primary or essential. The major significant causes of secondary hypertension in the elderly are intrinsic renal diseases and renovascular disease.

TABLE 5.2.   Recommended Diagnostic Tests for Hypertension in the Elderly

IN ALL PATIENTS
Urine analysis

Complete blood cell count (CBC)

Chemistry panels, including measurements of blood urea nitrogen (BUN), creatinine, electrolytes, uric acid, and lipids (with separate quantitation of high-density lipoprotein [HDL]).

Fasting serum glucose

A baseline electroencephalogram (ECG) to assess heart rate, axis, and degree of left

A baseline plain chest film to evaluate heart size and contour.

IN SELECTED PATIENTS
Creatinine clearance

Microalbuminemia

Serum calcium

Thyroid-stimulating hormone (TSH)

Fasting triglycerides

24-hour urinary protein

Glycosylated hemoglobin

TABLE 5.3.   Clues to Secondary Hypertension

Clue	Etiology
Abdominal bruit	Renovascular disease
Increased creatinine (serum); albuminuria	Renal parenchymal disease
Labile hypertension	Pheochromocytoma
Headaches, palpitations, perspiration	Pheochromocytoma
Abdominal or flank masses	Polycystic kidney
Truncal obesity with purple striae	Cushing's syndrome
Hypokalemia of unknown cause	Primary aldosteronism
Hypercalcemia	Hypoparathyroidism

Renovascular hypertension is an illness that occurs with increasing frequency in the aged. It presents with rapid worsening of preexisting hypotension or the new onset of moderate to severe hypertension. Pheochromocytomas, hypercortisolism, or primary hyperaldosteronism are very rare in this population.

WHEN TO REFER

Though the patient with hypertension rarely requires referral, the family physician should consider referring patients in the following situations:

• Renovascular hypertension present
• Hypertension not controlled with standard treatment
• Other unusual cause found for secondary hypertension

MANAGEMENT

General Principles

The benefit to treating diastolic hypertension is significant reduction in cardiovascular and stroke events. Treating isolated systolic hypertension also appears to reduce morbidity and mortality, but hypotension is a more common complication. The standard goals of hypertension treatment are to reduce the systolic pressure to less than 140 mm Hg and the diastolic pressure to less than 90 mm Hg. An intermediate goal of systolic blood pressure below 160 mm Hg may be appropriate in patients with marked systolic hypertension. Although these figures still hold in the elderly, it is important to be wary of the increased risks of therapy in this group. The goal of antihypertensive therapy should be to reduce morbidity and mortality without adversely affecting the patient's quality of life or functional abilities. This goal can be achieved by lifestyle modification alone or, if inadequate, with pharmacologic treatment.

It is common for the family physician to see patients diagnosed previously who have already begun taking antihypertensive medicines. If there is minimal to no evidence of end-organ damage, the diagnosis in these patients needs to be reevaluated. Often, when antihypertensives are withdrawn, the patient will remain normotensive.

A general approach to the treatment of hypertension is shown in Figure 5.1.

Nonpharmacologic Approaches

The nonpharmacologic approach can be used alone in patients with mild to moderate hypertension, thereby avoiding any medication-induced side effects. However, like younger hypertensives, many elderly patients are unable to maintain lifestyle changes and will require drug therapy. Usually, a 6-month to 1-year trial will separate those who require drug therapy from those whose blood pressure can be lowered without medications. If medication is

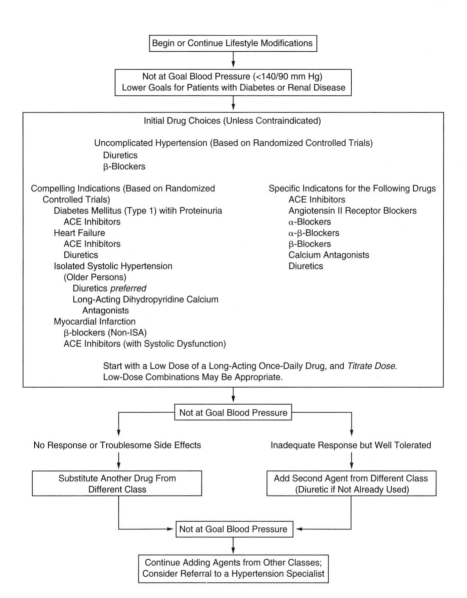

FIGURE 5.1. Algorithm for the treatment of hypertension. *ACE,* angiotensin-converting enzyme; *ISA,* intrinsic sympathomimetic activity. (Reprinted from the sixth report of the Joint National Committee on Prevention, Detection, Evaluation, and Treatment of High Blood Pressure. Arch Intern Med 1997;157:2430.)

required, nonpharmacologic interventions should still be continued. The following lifestyle changes should be recommended to patients:

- Weight loss
- Exercise
- Alcohol limitation
- Smoking cessation
- Limit sodium intake
- Maintain adequate potassium intake (caution in patients receiving angiotensin-converting enzyme [ACE] inhibitors)
- Decrease dietary fat

Pharmacotherapy

Only two agents have been shown to reduce hypertension-associated morbidity and mortality in older adults: diuretics and β-blockers (Table 5.4). The Joint National Committee on Prevention, Detection, Evaluation and Treatment of High Blood Pressure (JNC-VI) recommends that initial therapy in the elderly, unless contraindicated, be with one of these two classes of medications. In older persons with isolated systolic hypertension, diuretics have been shown to significantly improve morbidity. A more complicated approach is to evaluate coexisting disease states and choose an antihypertensive that will also exert an effect on these conditions. By applying this method, not only is blood pressure controlled, but therapy is being given for other underlying diseases. This approach also underscores understanding the beneficial and deleterious effects of various medications. Whichever approach is taken, some general information about prescribing antihypertensives for the elderly should be remembered:

- Begin therapy with a reduced drug dosage.
- Titrate therapy more slowly, increasing drug dosages no more frequently than every 2 to 4 weeks.
- Titrate drugs to maximally tolerated doses before initiating a second agent.
- Switch to another agent rather than adding a second drug.
- It may take months to adequately control hypertension while avoiding side-effects.
- Compliance is enhanced by once-daily dosing.

Diuretics

Diuretics are the most commonly used, initial antihypertensive agent in the elderly and have been clearly shown to reduce morbidity and mortality. This stems from three major factors:

- Proven efficacy
- Ease of administration (one pill a day)
- Low cost

TABLE 5.4. Oral Antihypertensive Drugs Commonly Used for Initial Management of Hypertension in the Elderly

Drug	Recommended Use	Usual Dose Range, Total mg/d[a] (Frequency per Day)	Selected Side Effects and Comments
Diuretics			Short term: increases cholesterol and glucose levels; biochemical abnormalities; decreases potassium, sodium, and magnesium levels, increases uric acid and calcium levels; rare: blood dyscrasias, photosensitivity, pancreatitis, hyponatremia
Chlorthalidone (Hygroton) (G)‡	Systolic heart failure	12.5 to 50 (1)	
Hydrochlorothiazide (Esidix) (G)		12.5 to 50 (1)	
Indapamide (Lozol)	Systolic and diastolic hypertension	1.25 to 5 (1)	(less or no hypercholesterolemia)
Metolazone (Diulo)		0.5 to 1.0 (1)	
Potassium-sparing agents			Hyperkalemia
Amiloride hydrochloride (Midamor) (G)		5 to 10 (1)	
Spironolactone (Aldactone) (G)		25 to 100 (1)	(Gynecomastia)
Triamterene (Dyrenium) (G)		25 to 100 (1)	
Alpha blockers			Postural hypotension
Doxazosin mesylate (Cardura) (G)		1 to 16 (1)	
Prazosin hydrochloride (Minipress) (G)		2 to 30 (2 to 3)	

continued

TABLE 5.4. *continued*

Drug	Recommended Use	Usual Dose Range, Total mg/d[a] (Frequency per Day)	Selected Side Effects and Comments
Terazosin hydrochloride (Hytrin)		1 to 20 (1)	
β-**Blockers**	Previous myocardial infarction; angina; diastolic heart failure		Bronchospasm, bradycardia, heart failure, may mask insulin-induced hypoglycemia; less serious: impaired peripheral circulation, insomnia, fatigue, decreased exercise tolerance, hypertriglyceridemia (except agents with intrinsic sympathomimetic activity)
Atenolol (Tenormin) (G)§		25–100 (1 to 2)	
Metoprolol tartrate (Lopressor) (G)§		50 to 300 (2)	
Metoprolol succinate (Toprol-XL)§		50–300 (1)	
Calcium antagonists			
Nondihydropyridines			Conduction defects, worsening of systolic dysfunction, gingival hyperplasia
Diltiazem hydrochloride (Cardizem SR)		120 to 360 (2)	(Nausea, headache)
Dihydropyridines			Edema of the ankle, flushing, headache, gingival hypertrophy
Amlodipine besylate (Norvasc)		2.5 to 10 (1)	
Nifedipine (Procardia XL)		30 to 120 (1)	
Angiotensin-converting enzyme inhibitors			Common: cough; rare: angioedema, hyperkalemia, rash, loss of taste, leukopenia

continued

TABLE 5.4. *continued*

Drug	Recommended Use	Usual Dose Range, Total mg/d*a* (Frequency per Day)	Selected Side Effects and Comments
Benazepril hydrochloride (Lotensin)		5 to 40 (1 to 2)	May worsen preexisting renal insufficiency
Captopril (Capoten) (G)		25 to 150 (2 to 3)	
Enalapril maleate (Vasotec)		5 to 40 (1 to 2)	
Fosinopril sodium (Monopril)		10 to 40 (1 to 2)	
Lisinopril (Zestril)		5 to 40 (1)	
Angiotensin II receptor blockers			Angioedema (very rare), hyperkalemia
Losartan potassium (Cozaar)		25 to 100 (1 to 2)	
Valsartan (Diovan)		80 to 320 (1)	
Irbesartan (Avapro)		150 to 300 (1)	

Adapted from Sixth Report of the Joint National Committee on Prevention, Detection, Evaluation, and Treatment of High Blood Pressure. Arch Intern Med 1997;157:2426.

*a*These dosages may vary from those listed in the Physicians Desk Reference 51st edition, which may be consulted for additional information. The listing of side effects is not all-inclusive, and side effects are for the class of drugs except where noted for individual drug (in parentheses); clinicians are urged to refer to the package insert for a more detailed listing.

G = Indicates generic available; ‡ = also acts centrally; § = cardioselective.

Diuretics also have a reasonably low side-effect profile. However, they can cause life-threatening hyponatremia (and hypokalemia or hyperkalemia) and dehydration in some frail elders and can lead to elevations in cholesterol, glucose, and uric acid and a reduced glomerular filtration rate. The majority of studies have been with chlorthalidone (Hygroton) and hydrochlorothiazide (Esidrix). The dosages used have been 12.5 to 50 mg a day, and pharmacologic data indicate that higher doses provide no further benefit to the patient. Rarely is there benefit from dosages greater than 25 mg. Other diuretics in common use are the potassium-sparing amiloride (Midamor) or spironolactone (Aldactone) and combinations of a thiazide and a potassium-sparing diuretic. There have been no studies of these agents in treating hypertension in the elderly. The more potent loop diuretics such as furosemide (Lasix) or metolazone (Diulo) have no role in uncomplicated antihypertensive therapy.

β-Blockers

β-Blockers are also antihypertensives with proven efficacy. They should be considered first-line agents in the elderly and are particularly effective in patients with a history of atherosclerotic heart disease, angina, diastolic heart failure, and previous myocardial infarctions. In these patients there is a decrease in myocardial contractility and heart rate, which reduces myocardial oxygen demand and thereby reduces ischemic events. However, because of contraindications, β-blockers either should not be used or should be used with great caution in elderly patients with the following conditions:

• Systolic heart failure (because of the negative effect of β-blockers on myocardial contractility)
• Bradycardias or sick sinus syndrome (because of the negative inotropic effects of β-blockers)
• COPD, peripheral vascular disease, or diabetes (because of the serious drug-related problems with β-blockers)

The less lipophilic β-blockers are preferred because their entry into the central nervous system is diminished. The common side effects of all classes of β-blockers are fatigue/lethargy, decline in mental status, and a slowing of the heart rate.

ACE Inhibitors

ACE inhibitors have a distinct advantage in the treatment of elderly hypertensive patients who have heart failure and left ventricular hypertrophy. They may also have a role in the treatment of patients with glucose and lipid metabolism problems because they do not alter glucose and lipid metabolism.

ACE inhibitors have not been well studied in the elderly and therefore are believed by some physicians to be second-line agents in the treatment of routine hypertension. However, because of their relatively low side-effect profile, with minimal central nervous system or metabolic problems, they are a frequent choice in the elderly. ACE inhibitors have been shown to be of benefit to renal function early on in diabetic patients by reducing proteins through positive renovascular effects. They are gaining more widespread use in elderly patients with non–insulin-dependent diabetes mellitus (NIDDM) who have any evidence of proteinuria.

The use of ACE inhibitors in older adults is limited by the renal effects of these medications. Significant hyperkalemia and renal insufficiency occur more commonly in older adults on ACE inhibitors. Close monitoring of serum potassium and serum creatinine levels is necessary, and medication must be discontinued if abnormalities are detected. Fortunately, with close observation, these agents rarely produce frank renal failure. In some patients the use of ACE inhibitors is limited by the development of a nonproductive cough, a rash, or, rarely, angioneurotic edema.

Calcium Channel Blockers
Calcium channel blockers, also called calcium antagonists, are used to treat hypertension in the elderly. As with ACE inhibitors, many physicians do not consider them first-line agents. However, they are particularly good agents for patients with angina and peripheral vascular disease. There are significant changes in the clearance of these drugs in older adults so that smaller or less frequent doses can be utilized. Calcium antagonists are best thought of in three classes:

- Phenylalkylamines
- Dihydropyridines
- Benzothiazepines

Phenylalkylamines have the most negative inotropic and chronotropic effects, causing a worsening ejection fraction and a decrease in heart rate. Drugs in this group such as verapamil (Calan) should not be used in patients with heart failure or heart block. In addition, verapamil is associated with significant constipation from smooth-muscle effects within the gastrointestinal tract.

Dihydropyridines (e.g., nifedipine [Procardia]) have the most potent effect on the peripheral vascular system, causing vasodilatation. They are the most likely to lead to peripheral edema, hypotension, and reflex tachycardia.

Benzothiazepines (e.g., diltiazem [Cardizem]) have effects similar to but less than both the other classes of calcium agonists.

Other Agents
Probably the best of these other agents used in the elderly, with good effects on reduction of blood pressure, are the α-adrenergic receptor antagonists such as terazosin (Hytrin) or doxazosin (Cardura). These agents are potent vasodilators and can cause significant orthostatic hypotension. However, they have been shown to improve urinary flow in patients with prostatic obstruction, a common complaint in elderly men. The use of low doses (2.5 to 5 mg) of these medications given at bedtime can have a beneficial effect on both blood pressure and the symptoms of prostatism. Centrally acting α-agonists such as clonidine (Catapres) are rarely used because of their side effects on the central nervous system with the accompanying cognitive changes. The transdermal delivery system has found a niche in patients who

cannot swallow medications, although the central nervous system effects of sedation and/or confusion must be monitored carefully.

Agents such as methyldopa (Aldomet) and reserpine (Serpasil) have been used effectively in the past as second-line agents in elderly hypertensive studies. They are of limited use at present because of concerns about side effects and because of the beneficial effects of newer agents.

Appropriate medication choices can be affected by coexisting medical conditions (Table 5.5). A second drug can be added if the initial medication choice is inadequate. Diuretics are a good second-stop agent if not used initially. Multidrug therapy is becoming more common for good control.

Complications with Drug Therapy

In most elderly patients a reduction in systolic pressure to 160 mm Hg will be the goal. Some frail elders with significant systolic hypertension cannot tolerate this pressure secondary to medication side effects and low blood pressures, causing low perfusion of the central nervous system. In these cases the physician should settle for reductions to 180 mm Hg. Remember, the patient is not best served if his or her functional abilities are impaired in an attempt to lower the blood pressure to reduce future morbidity or mortality.

TABLE 5.5. Guidelines for Choosing Initial Drugs for Essential Hypertension Drug

	CAD	CHF	LVH	Decreased HR	DM	COPD	Gout	Increased lipids	CRI
Diuretics									
Thiazide	—	Yes	—	—	—	—	No	No	No
Loop	—	Yes	—	—	—	—	No	—	Yes
Potassium sparing	—	—	—	—	—	—	—	—	No
β-Blockers	Yes	No	—	No	—	No	—	No	—
α-Blockers	—	—	—	Yes	Yes	—	—	Yes	—
ACE Inhibitors	Yes	Yes	—	Yes	Yes	—	—	—	Yes
Calcium blockers									
Diltiazem	—	No	—	No	Yes	—	—	—	Yes
Verapamil	—	No	—	No	Yes	—	—	—	Yes
Dihydropyridines	—	—	—	—	Yes	—	—	—	Yes
α₂ agonist									
Methyldopa	—	—	—	Yes	—	—	—	—	—

Adapted from Taylor RB. Manual of family practice. Boston: Little, Brown, pp. 274–275.

Note: Either a thiazide diuretic or a β-blocker is recommended if coexisting conditions do not suggest otherwise.

Yes = drug is preferred; No = drug is relatively contraindicated; — = drug acceptable; evidence insufficient to rank treatment options. ACE = angiotensin-converting enzyme; CAD = coronary artery disease; CHF = congestive heart failure; LVH = left ventricular hypertrophy; decreased HR = bradycardia; DM = diabetes mellitus; COPD = chronic obstructive pulmonary disease; increased lipids = dyslipidemia; CRI = chronic renal insufficiency.

Orthostatic hypotension is the most common complication with antihypertensive medication. Orthostasis can manifest as dizziness, falls, or as more vague symptoms such as weakness and fatigue. Other common concerns with antihypertensives include effects on sexual function, mood, and cognitive abilities.

FOLLOW-UP

In monitoring the course of hypertensive disease, the following should be observed:

- Hypertension is one of the classic medical illnesses where follow-up visits are key.
- Patients should be seen within 1 to 2 months after the initiation of therapy.
- After control is established, follow-up can be done at 3-month to 6-month intervals.
- Blood pressure monitoring in older adults should be performed standing as well as sitting to recognize postural hypotension. Also, if standing blood pressures are consistently lower than those sitting, the standing blood pressure should be used to regulate medication dosages.
- Patients are usually asymptomatic, and their treatment plan is for long-term therapy.
- Effective follow-up reinforces the message that compliance with medication is essential to reduce morbidity and mortality.

Initially the patient should be followed with frequent visits to ensure adequacy of the response to lifestyle modification or the chosen nonpharmacologic treatment. The beneficial effects of lifestyle changes should occur in 6 months to 1 year. If no benefit is observed, patients should be started on antihypertensive medications.

Follow-up laboratory testing depends on the particular agent chosen, but in general most elderly hypertensives should have an annual EKG and at least annual measurements of electrolytes and creatinine levels.

It is appropriate to consider withdrawing antihypertensive therapy from some patients after more than 1 year. Elderly patients who make lifestyle changes or who experience intercurrent illnesses may be normotensive when they are not receiving this medication. When elderly patients require hospitalization or move into a more dependent living arrangement, they should be reevaluated for the continued use of all chronic medications. The physician should take an elderly person off a drug if its benefit has waned or its risk has increased.

PATIENT EDUCATION

The following are key areas to cover with patients:

- High blood pressure is not an inevitable result of the aging process.

- Patients with hypertension who are adequately treated may still have higher vascular risk than patients without hypertension. Good blood pressure control does not mean just lowering blood pressure to normal level.
- Adherence to the medication regimen is important. Both verbal and written instructions should be included. Blood pressure medication compliance can be enhanced in the elderly with some type of reminder system. A pillbox, a calendar pill system, a monthly blister pack, or some local creation may mean the difference between correct and incorrect dosing.
- Identification of a supportive individual who can offer reinforcement is helpful.

Suggested readings

Applegate WB, Rutan GH. Advances in management of hypertension in older persons. J Am Geriatr Soc 1992;40:1164-1174.

Insua JT, Sacks HS, Lau TS, et al. Drug treatment of hypertension in the elderly: a meta analysis. Ann Intern Med 1994;121:355-362.

Joint National Committee on Prevention, Detection, Evaluation and Treatment of High Blood Pressure: the sixth report. Arch Intern Med 1997;157:2401-2402.

Meuser D. Hypertension. In: Ham R, Sloane PD, eds. Primary care geriatrics. St. Louis: Mosby-Yearbook, 1997:561-576

National High Blood Pressure Education Program working report on hypertension in the elderly. Hypertension 1994;23:275-285

The Systolic Hypertension in the Elderly Program (SHEP) Cooperative Research Group. Prevention of stroke by antihypertensive drug treatment in older patients with isolated systolic hypertension: final results of SHEP. JAMA 1991;265:3255-3264.

CHAPTER 6

Osteoarthritis

Osteoarthritis, also known as degenerative joint disease, is the most common form of arthritis in the elderly. It occurs in up to 40% of people over age 65. Osteoarthritis is a dynamic condition that involves the simultaneous and progressive breakdown and repair of articular cartilage. The exact cause is unknown, but alteration in cartilage on both a biochemical and a structural level is involved. Joint injury, repetitive trauma, genetics, hormones, immune functions, obesity, and aging all contribute to the development of clinical joint disease.

The development of the cartilaginous degeneration occurs because of the poor healing properties of this tissue. Damage to the cartilage from even minimal trauma results in injuries that are not repaired and that accumulate with aging. The longer one lives with repeated trauma, the more degeneration that occurs. Osteoarthritis becomes a slowly progressive disease that results in loss of articular cartilage and destruction of the bony surfaces of the joint.

Osteoarthritis can be classified as idiopathic/primary or secondary to distinguish underlying pathophysiology (Table 6.1).

CHIEF COMPLAINT

Joint pain, which becomes increasingly severe as the disease progresses, is the chief complaint. Other complaints may include the following:

- Stiffness that usually occurs in the morning or after periods of inactivity and lasts less than 30 minutes in duration. This "gelling" phenomenon, caused by an increase in the viscosity of synovial fluid secondary to increased proteoglycans resulting from cartilage breakdown, usually clears with a few minutes of motion. Gelling stiffness occurs commonly in the knees and hips after prolonged sitting and causes the patient to have difficulty arising and initiating his first steps. It is also common to have gelling stiffness after kneeling such as while gardening.
- Redness and swelling. These dual complaints accompany the body's inflammatory response and occur only occasionally in patients with osteoarthritis.

TABLE 6.1. Secondary Causes of Osteoarthritis

METABOLIC
Wilson's disease (defective copper metabolism, resulting in accumulation of copper in liver, brain, kidney, cornea, and other tissues)
Gaucher's disease

ENDOCRINE
Hyperparathyroidism
Diabetes mellitus
Hypothyroidism

NEUROPATHIC
Charcot joints

CONGENITAL
Legg-Calve Perthes disease (osteochrondrosis of the capitular epiphysis of the femur)
Congenital hip dislocation

EPIDEMIOLOGIC CONSIDERATIONS

- Osteoarthritis is the most common chronic condition in the elderly, occurring in more than 50% of the population over the age of 65.
- Some of the risk factors include obesity and participation in repetitive traumatic activities such as certain sports or occupations.
- It is familial, though not a specific inherited pattern.

- Abnormal lumps and or bumps in the hands and knees.
- "Giving way" sensation of the knee; hip pain causes a shift in gait to avoid bearing weight on the joint.
- Difficulty with activities of daily living such as opening doors and jars, going up and down stairs, and getting in and out of the bath or out of a chair.
- Joint motion causes sensations of popping, creaking, and pain and sounds of grinding with motion. Knees are most commonly affected; the distal interphalangeal (DIP) joint and posterior interphalangeal (PIP) joint are also affected.

HISTORY

The history is a key component in differentiating the various joint disease (Table 6.2). Osteoarthritis affects key joints, as noted above, and rarely involves the wrists elbows, ankles, or shoulders. In addition, patients with os-

TABLE 6.2.   Differential Diagnosis of Osteoarthritis

Disorder	Osteoarthritis	Rheumatoid Arthritis	Gout	Pseudogout	Polymyalgia Rheumatica	Joint Infection
HISTORICAL FEATURES						
Joint stiffness	++	++++	+	+	++	++
Joint pain	+++	+++	++++	++++	+	++++
Joint crepitus	+++	+	++	++	0	0
Fatigue/malaise	0	++	+	+	++++	+++
PHYSICAL FINDINGS						
Joint tenderness	++++	++++	+++++	+++++	+	++++
Joint erythema and warmth	+	++++	++++	++++	+	++++
Joint swelling	+++	++++	++++	++++	+	++++
Symmetrical joint involvement	+	+++	+	+	++++	0
Muscle tenderness	+	+	+	+	++++	0
Nonjoint findings	0	++	+	+	++++	++++
DIP and PIP joints involved	++++	+	++	++	+	+
Wrist involvement	+	++++	+	+	+	+
LABORATORY FINDINGS						
Synovial fluid	Minimal WBCs; normal viscosity	Viscous; many WBCs	Crystals; (negatively birefringent)	Crystals; (positively birefringent)	Normal	Viscous; WBCs
Elevated peripheral WBC	0	+	0	0	0	+++
Elevated ESR	0	+++	+	+	+++	++++
Anemia	0	++	0	0	+++	0
RADIOGRAPHIC FINDINGS						
	Joint asymmetry; bony sclerosis; subchondral cysts	Joint destruction; bony erosions; periarticular osteoporosis	Joint destruction; tophi bony erosions with sclerotic margins	Calcium deposition; chondrocalcinosis	Normal	Bone destruction

TABLE 6.3. Common Symptoms of Osteoarthritis at Specific Sites

Site	Complaints in Early Disease	Complaints in Late Disease
Small joints of hands	Stiffness, pain with motion, swelling, tenderness, crepitus	Heberden's nodes (bony enlargement of DIP joint) Bouchard's nodes (bony enlargement of PIP joints) Deformity and deviation in joints Decreased limitation of movement
Hips	Groin/thigh pain Difficulty walking secondary to stiffness or pain Unilateral or bilateral	Inability to fully extend hip—contractures Abnormal gait Pain at rest Hip abnormally rotated
Knees	Pain, stiffness, gelling, tenderness, swelling, crepitus	Bony hypertrophy (lumps, bumps around joint) Deformity and deviation of joint Inability to fully extend or flex
Spine	Back pain, stiffness Lack of full range of motion—flexion, extension, rotation	Severe pain with motion Loss of range of motion Nerve root impingement causing pain into buttocks or down the leg Distal motor/sensory changes

teoarthritis rarely complain of systemic illness or nonjoint symptoms such as fever, malaise, or weight loss.

The pain of osteoarthritis is worse with activity, particularly weight-bearing activity that increases the bone-to-bone joint contact. Pain is intermittent in early disease and constant in late disease. Pain is usually relieved with rest, although late in the disease pain can be severe with little activity. Various joints can be involved (Table 6.3).

Symptoms of the hip may be perceived as unilateral or bilateral groin pain. Frequently, such pain can be referred to the buttocks or lateral thigh.

Osteoarthritis of the spine begins as aches and pains, but can lead to narrowing of the joint spaces and neuroforamina. Spinal symptoms then relate to nerve compression and referred pain down the nerve distribution, which can present as the following:

- Shoulder, arm, or hand pain in the cervical spine
- Sciatic-type symptoms in the lumbar spine

Within the spine, severe osteoarthritic changes can lead to blockage of the spinal canal and spinal stenosis syndrome. This syndrome is increasing in frequency among the elderly as more persons are living longer with osteoarthritic changes. Spinal stenosis is characterized by the following:

- Back and leg pain are present.
- Decreased urinary and/or rectal sphincter tone is present.
- The pain worsens with walking and prolonged standing, but is relieved with rest and position changes that flex the lumbar spine.
- The patient may walk or stand in a stooped position to alleviate the pain.

PHYSICAL EXAMINATION

The physical findings of osteoarthritis are limited to the affected joints and the neuromuscular changes that result from the joint disease. Bone and joint findings may include the following:

- Joint tenderness.
- Joint pain, with both active and passive range of motion. The joints involved are characteristically the knees, hips, cervical and lumbar sacral spine, DIP and PIP joints, respectively, and the first carpal-metacarpal joint.
- Joint crepitus. Damaged cartilage and bony changes can create vibrations with motion that are sensed by the patient and can be felt from surface palpation. Crepitus is incorrectly seen as representing loose intraarticular impediments. It usually results from inflammatory changes within the cartilage, causing nodule formation or surface irregularities that catch and give way with movement.
- Bony deformity. The knees and hand joints affected by osteoarthritis develop bony changes that create abnormal structural features such as Heberden's nodes in the DIP joints of the hands and Bouchard's nodes in the PIP joints of the hands.
- Bony hypertrophy. Heberden's and Bouchard's nodes.
- Minimal signs of acute inflammation. Redness and swelling are present early in the disease and become more common as the cartilage breakdown and bony damage lead to an increased inflammatory reaction. Increased pain, redness, and swelling can also occur with bleeding into the joint, which occurs with progression of joint damage.
- Loss of motion. Joints damaged by degenerative changes lose motion secondary to pain, inflammation, and bony changes. This loss is significant for it affects the patient's functional abilities. Lack of flexion and rotation in the spine, hips, and knees leads to significant gait instability.
- Vagus or varus deformities of the knee joint.
- Gait instabilities.

Muscle findings may include atrophy, which can result from inactivity or neurologic impingement.

Neurologic findings related to osteoarthritic changes in the spine may include nerve root damage or resultant neurologic changes in the distribution of those nerves.

Diagnostic test data

Laboratory tests may be extremely helpful in distinguishing among rheumatologic disorders, as well as in planning therapy. (See Table 6.2 for the differential diagnosis of osteoarthritis.)

Blood Tests

There are no specific blood tests for diagnosing osteoarthritis; in fact most tests are normal. Blood test abnormalities are more common with other rheumatic conditions and may be definitive (see Table 6.2). An increased incidence of false-positive autoantibodies in the elderly or a positive rheumatoid factor or antinuclear antibody test is not uncommon. Elevated uric acid levels occur with aging and some common medications and should not sway one away from the diagnosis of osteoarthritis.

Chemistry panels to evaluate renal and hepatic function are important in planning and monitoring therapy.

Radiologic Tests

Though plain-film radiographs are not necessary to make the diagnosis of osteoarthritis, they can confirm the diagnosis and differentiate osteoarthritis from other diseases. Radiographic findings roughly correlate with clinical symptoms (Table 6.4).

TABLE 6.4.   Radiographic Changes in Osteoarthritis

Disease Stage	Films	Clinical Symptoms
Very early disease	Normal	Pain, stiffness
Early disease	Joint-space narrowing Bony sclerosis Subchondral cysts Developing osteophytes Bone spurring Bone deformities and decreasing motion	Pain, stiffness, swelling
Late disease	Gross deformity, joint deviation Breakdown of bone surfaces Loss of joint space	Contractures Lack of motion Pain at rest

- Most patients will get x-rays early to rule out fracture or tumor.
- Early in the disease, when the pathologic process has affected only the cartilaginous tissues, plain films will be normal.
- As the disease progresses, plain films will begin to show asymmetric, joint-space narrowing and subchondral reactive sclerosis.
- In more advanced disease, subchondral cysts, osteophytes, bony deformities, and subluxations can be seen.

Joint Fluid Aspiration

Aspiration of the joint fluid is necessary to eliminate other diagnoses such as infection, gout, or pseudogout, especially with acute joint swelling, redness, and pain. In patients with osteoarthritis the following occur:

- The joint fluid is usually a noninflammatory translucent liquid.
- The viscosity is normal.
- The mucin clot is firm.
- The cell count is only slightly elevated (<2000 white blood cells).
- There are occasional crystals of hydroxyapatite in the synovial fluid from the destruction of the cartilage.

WHEN TO REFER

It may be necessary to refer a patient for an unclear diagnosis. Patients with osteoarthritis generally benefit from referrals to physical and occupational therapists for muscle strengthening, joint protection, and gait evaluations. Also, physical and occupational therapy can help the patient in performing activities of daily living.

Some patients will require surgical intervention, usually by orthopedic surgeons. Intervention includes arthroscopic and open-joint procedures for both soft-tissue and bony changes or total joint replacement when the joint is so badly damaged that arthroscopy or joint replacement is necessary.

MANAGEMENT

Figure 6.1 presents an algorithm for management of osteoarthritis. The following are the goals of management of osteoarthritis:

- Adequate pain relief
- Decreasing ongoing joint destruction, as evidenced by diminished pain and better mobility
- Maximizing the patient's functional abilities
- Determining the patient's functional abilities guides and monitors therapy. Understanding how the joint disease affects a patient's abilities to perform the basic and instrumental activities of daily living will help guide treatment.

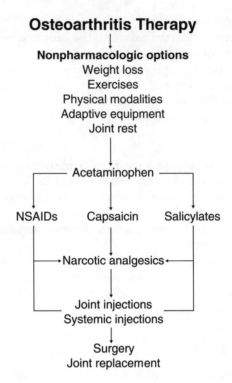

Osteoarthritis Therapy
↓
Nonpharmacologic options
Weight loss
Exercises
Physical modalities
Adaptive equipment
Joint rest
↓
Acetaminophen
NSAIDs   Capsaicin   Salicylates
→Narcotic analgesics←
Joint injections
Systemic injections
↓
Surgery
Joint replacement

FIGURE 6.1. Algorithm for management of osteoarthritis.

These goals require a combined approach using the following:

- Nonpharmacologic interventions
- Medications
- Surgery

Nonpharmacologic Interventions

Daily Rest and Joint Protection

Modifications of the patient's daily life to increase periods of joint rest are beneficial to the preservation of joint function. Protecting joints by avoiding repetitive trauma or joint stress will also preserve joint function. Classic teaching about resting a painful joint is a two-edged sword in the older adult with osteoarthritis. Joint rest with or without immobilization or splinting can decrease pain and inflammation. However, joint inactivity will quickly lead to increased stiffness, atrophy of muscles, and decreased range of motion. Therefore joint rest should be kept to a minimum (15 to 30 minutes, three to four times daily), and range of motion exercises encouraged. For severe pain, rest periods of no more than 24 hours are best.

Weight Loss

It is essential to reduce the ongoing damage to the weight-bearing joints by reducing body mass and/or weight, which will result in a noticeable reduction in pain.

Exercise

A well-designed exercise program focused on strengthening the periarticular musculature and maintaining range of motion will benefit all patients with osteoarthritis. The best exercises minimize both the forces across the joints and repetitive joint motion. Aquatic exercises are well tolerated and helpful. Supine exercises are the most beneficial for the spine. A well-trained physical therapist can guide the patient with a useful exercise program depending on the specific joints affected. Poor exercise plans can lead to more joint damage and greater pain by traumatizing cartilage. Running, jumping, and weight-lifting are all poor choices for patients with osteoarthritis.

Physical Modalities

Pain relief can be achieved using one or more of the following physical modalities either by the patient at home or under the direction of rehabilitation personnel:

- Local heat therapy
- Ultrasound
- Diathermy
- Paraffin baths
- Transcutaneous electrical nerve stimulators (for patients with osteoarthritis of the spine)

Adaptive Equipment

Patients with osteoarthritis should be counseled about the use of adaptive equipment for joint protection, pain relief, and gait stability. Physical and occupational therapists are excellent resources for information about this equipment. Some examples of adaptive equipment include orthotics for the feet, jar openers, cooking utensils, special canes, walkers, splints, and braces. Most insurance plans reimburse for these items.

Medications

Topical

Topical medications, such as capsaicin (Zostrix), for joint pain have been shown to be effective. Capsaicin acts by altering neuropeptide levels in the peripheral nervous system and decreasing neurotransmission. It requires a few days of application to the skin overlying the affected joint before any relief can be expected and is of particular benefit in knee and finger-joint pain.

Oral

Oral agents for the treatment of osteoarthritis are probably more effective in reducing pain than in halting joint destruction. This is in contrast to therapy for other rheumatologic conditions in which decreasing inflammation and altering the disease process is the primary goal. The following are the medications most commonly used for osteoarthritis:

- Acetaminophen
- Nonsteroidal, antiinflammatory drugs (NSAIDs)
- Salicylates (to a limited extent)
- Opioids (only in selected patients)

Acetaminophen is the agent of choice for most patients with osteoarthritis. The risk for toxicity is low, with a maximum dose of 1000 mg four times daily. However, patients with liver disease should not receive such a large dose. It has been shown to be as effective in relieving osteoarthritis pain as NSAIDs and has a much lower incidence of side effects. It may be supplemented with other analgesics if necessary. The following are examples:

- Ibuprofen (Motrin), 200 to 800 mg, three to four times daily
- Indomethacin (Indocin), 25 to 50 mg, three to four times daily
- Naproxen (Naprosyn), 250 to 750 mg, two times daily
- Sulindac (Clinoril), 150 to 200 mg, two times daily

NSAIDs have been the mainstay of therapy for many years and are only being replaced by acetaminophen because of toxicity. They are highly effective pain relievers and work very well to decrease inflammation of the osteoarthritic joint. However, NSAIDs have a high incidence of serious side effects—gastrointestinal bleeding, dyspepsia, renal damage, hepatotoxicity, and sodium retention—which occur at a higher rate in the elderly, and their usefulness is therefore limited in this population. Misoprostol (Cytotec) is sometimes prescribed in combination with NSAIDs to reduce gastrointestinal side effects. However, the cost and side effects of misoprostol itself have limited the use of this combination.

Salicylates, the original agents for treating osteoarthritis pain, still have a limited role in current therapy. Like NSAIDs, they are effective pain relievers, yet their use is limited because of gastrointestinal toxicity and antiplatelet effects. Enteric-coated aspirins or nonacetylated salicylic acids, up to 2000 mg per day, cause less gastrointestinal upset and are used in some patients.

Opioids are the most potent analgesics and should be used in patients in whom adequate relief is not obtained from other modalities. The most commonly used drugs in this class are codeine, hydrocodone, and oxycodone.

The decision to use opioids must weigh the risk of tolerance and addiction (with long-term use) against the severity of pain and how much it interferes with daily function and quality of life.

Parenteral Therapy

The use of intraarticular steroid injections can result in dramatic response in selected patients. The most common uses are for the following:

- Acute flares of single joints
- Joint pain unresponsive to multiple medications
- When one or two joints are causing limitation in functional abilities

The following joints are the most commonly accessible for injection:

- Knee joints
- Metacarpal phalangeal joints
- Spinal articulations (occasionally)

The steroid is mixed with a locally acting anesthetic (bupivacaine [Marcaine], lidocaine [Xylocaine]) and injected into the joint space. The anesthetic will produce almost immediate pain reduction and within 24 hours the steroid will begin to decrease inflammation and pain. Pain reduction typically lasts for months, and repeat injections can be given up to three to four times a year.

Steroid joint injection therapy is administered as follows:

- Mix steroid with anesthetic such as lidocaine
- Volume injected depends on joint
  - Small joints = 0.5 to 1 mL
  - Large joints = 5 to 10 mL

Some patients may experience a flare during first 24 to 48 hours after injection.

The most commonly used steroid preparations are listed in Table 6.5. The dosage and administration of intraarticular steroids depends on the joint being injected (Table 6.6). Although controversial, a single intramuscular injection of steroids used on the same frequency can relieve pain (Table 6.7).

Steroid use is complicated by the following, sometimes-serious side effects:

- Hyperglycemia
- Cataract development
- Myopathy
- Hypertension

TABLE 6.5. Commonly Used Steroid Preparations for Joint Injection

Preparation	Preparation Strength
Triamcinolones	
Hexacetonide (Aristospan)	20 mg/mL
Acetonide (Kenalog)	40 mg/mL
Diacetate (Aristocort)	40 mg/mL
Methylprednisolone acetate (Depo-Medrol)	20 mg/mL
	40 mg/mL
	80 mg/mL

TABLE 6.6. Administration of Steroids in the Treatment of Osteoarthritis

Joint	Lidocaine 1% Dose (mL)	Steroid Dose (mg)	Needle Size (Gauge and Length)
Small joints of hand	0.25 to 0.5	5 to 10	25 (1 in)
Shoulder	5	20 to 40	20 to 22 (1.5 in)
Knee	5	40 to 80	20 (1.5 in)

TABLE 6.7. Systemic Steroid Therapy for Osteoarthritis

Intramuscular Gluteal Injection	Dose
Methylprednisolone acetate (Depo-Medrol)	40 to 80 mg
Dexamethasone acetate (Decadron-La)	4 to 8 mg
Betamethasone acetate (Celestone Soluspan)	6 to 12 mg

Surgery

Surgery for patients with osteoarthritis should be considered when medical therapy has been unsuccessful in relieving joint pain, when joints are unstable, or when activities of daily living and quality of life are affected by pain or immobility. Surgery can remove osteophytes, which cause pain, impinge on nerves, and limit motion. Removal of loose cartilage or other soft-tissue fragments can improve pain and motion. Joint replacement can allow a patient with end-stage osteoarthritis to regain function. Surgical options include the following:

- Osteotomy for patients with osteoarthritis of the knee
- Arthroscopy for patients with knee involvement to remove debris, smooth cartilage, and irrigate the joint

- Joint replacements of the knee, hip, and, rarely, IP and MCP joints
- Prosthesis in weight-bearing joints (knees, hips), which lasts 15 to 20 years

Complications of surgery include deep venous thrombosis, pulmonary emboli, and joint infections. Long-term complications include infections and loosening of prosthesis. Patients with artificial joints require antibiotic prophylaxis with dental and other procedures associated with transient bacteremia.

PATIENT EDUCATION

The following are key points to convey to patients:

- Early diagnosis and treatment can help slow the progression of disabling joint damage.
- There is no cure for osteoarthritis.
- Physical therapy and/or exercise can lessen pain and improve flexibility and joint mobility.
- Applications of heat may make joints more mobile, while applications of cold reduce swelling and help relieve pain.
- Controlling body weight and avoiding injury can reduce the risk of osteoarthritis.
- Warm, dry climates may relieve symptoms.
- Remedies that sound too good to be true probably are.
- More information is available through the Arthritis Foundation (800-283-7800).

FOLLOW-UP

Osteoarthritis is a chronic condition that requires ongoing evaluation and management. A joint affected by osteoarthritis can develop a secondary problem. Osteoarthritic joints are more prone to infections than normal joints. Crystal-induced joint diseases can occur in patients with osteoarthritis. All joint flares should prompt an aspiration of the fluid for cell count, gram stain, culture, and microscopic exam for crystals.

Follow-up of the patient with osteoarthritis includes the following:

- Assessment of symptoms
- Assessment of pain control (if insufficient control, add or change medications; if sufficient, reduce chronic medications)
- Emphasis of nonpharmacologic options
- Weight loss
- Exercise
- Adaptive equipment

- Joint rest and protection
- Physical and occupational therapy
- Evaluation of new joint complaints—redness, swelling, increased pain
- Evaluation for joint infection—consider fluid aspiration for white blood cell (WBC) count
- Evaluation for new joint inflammation—consider fluid aspiration for crystal disease, acute bleeding
- Evaluation for disease progression
  - Need for adaptive equipment
  - Time for surgical evaluation
  - Evidence of osteoarthritis in the spine causing neurologic impingement or spinal stenosis

SUGGESTED READINGS

Hochberg M, Altman RD, Brandt KD. Guidelines for the management of osteoarthritis. Arthritis Rheum 1995;38:1535-1546.

Swedberg JA, Steinbauer JR. Osteoarthritis. Am Fam Phys 1992;45:557-568.

Puett DW, Griffin MR. Published trials of nonmedicinal and noninvasive therapies for hip and knee osteoarthritis. Ann Intern Med 1994;121:33-140.

Bradley JD, Brandt KD, Katz DP. Comparison of an antiinflammatory dose of ibuprofen, an analgesic dose of ibuprofen, and acetaminophen in the treatment of patients with osteoarthritis of the knee. N Engl J Med 1991;325:87-91.

CHAPTER 7
....

Parkinson's Disease

Parkinson's disease, a classic neurodegenerative disorder, occurs more commonly in elderly patients causing symptoms known as Parkinsonism, consisting of tremor, bradykinesia, and rigidity. There is little to offer therapeutically to alter the disease's progression, and treatments are directed toward symptom management. Symptoms are usually mild initially and become progressively worse. To complicate matters further, the presence of dual neurodegenerative diseases, particularly Alzheimer's and Parkinson's, is common in the elderly. Parkinsonism can also be secondary to certain metabolic disorders, a few other neurodegenerative syndromes, or exposure to neuroleptic drugs or certain neurotoxic substances.

Although many physicians think of Parkinson's disease as resulting from a loss of dopamine cells within the substantia nigra, the neurodegeneration is not confined to this single area of the brain. Patients with Parkinson's disease also exhibit neuron loss in the temporal and parietal lobes, resulting in a dementia-like syndrome. This pathologic process occurs in about 1% of persons over age 50. There are about 50,000 new cases of Parkinson's disease diagnosed per year in the United States. Onset typically occurs between the ages of 55 and 70, and men are affected slightly more often than women. Parkinson's disease occurs less frequently among persons of African-American and Japanese ancestry. The disease is not thought to be familial, although research in this area is ongoing.

CHIEF COMPLAINT

Patients vary in their tolerance for symptoms of Parkinsonism. Some will wait until the symptoms are relatively advanced before seeking treatment. Initial complaints may come from patients or a person close to them. Common chief complaints include the following:

- Tremor—hand shaking, one or both hands
- Gait difficulties
- Loss of balance/falls
- Bradykinesia (difficulty rising from chair, slow walking)

- Seborrhea (flaky, scaly skin in scalp, eyebrows)
- Sialorrhea (drooling, excessive saliva)
- Autonomic dysfunction
  - Temperature variations (hot, cold, sweaty, "goosebumps")
  - Dizziness and/or faintness with standing
  - Constipation, urinary incontinence/retention
  - Orthostasis
- Forgetfulness, loss of short-term memory (usually noted by family)

HISTORY

Parkinson's disease should be suspected in patients presenting with any of the above chief complaints. A careful history should be undertaken to search for other subtle symptoms. Because Parkinson's disease is a gradually progressive neurodegenerative disorder, symptoms are frequently not noticed by the patient or family until they are more severe. Early signs of bradykinesia, balance dysfunction, micrographia, sialorrhea, or seborrhea are often ignored.

A careful medication history is important. A variety of medications, including the phenothiazines, reserpine (Serpasil), methyldopa (Aldomet), metochlopramide (Reglan), and other dopamine antagonists, can cause early Parkinson-like changes. Evidence of metabolic disorder or exposure to other neurotoxic medication needs to be uncovered. The impact caused by the symptoms on activities of daily living will determine the treatment plan.

PHYSICAL EXAMINATION

The physical exam is key to the diagnosis of Parkinson's disease. The classic triad of Parkinson's disease includes the following:

- Tremor
- Bradykinesis
- Rigidity

Tremor

Tremor is the hallmark of Parkinson's disease. In fact, when James Parkinson wrote the initial treatise on the disease, he named it the "shaking palsy." Distinguishing between common tremors is crucial in making a correct diagnosis (Table 7.1).

Testing

The tremor should be tested for its response to motion. Hand or leg motion will make a Parkinson's tremor diminish in intensity, or at the worst, will have no effect on the tremor. In contrast, essential tremor is exacerbated with motion. Asymmetry of the tremor should be ascertained by asking the individ-

TABLE 7.1.   Differential Diagnosis of Tremor

Tremor (Pseudonyms)	Clinical Findings
Physiologic (nonpathologic)	Low amplitude and high frequency Aggravated by stress; caffeine, fatigue; medications, such as amphetamines, adrenergic agonists, and theophylline preparations Primarily occurs in hands Bilateral more often than unilateral Eliminated by alcohol ingestion
Essential tremor (familial tremor, intention tremor, benign tremor, senile tremor)	Most common pathologic tremor Increased prevalence with aging Varying amplitude but low frequency Bilateral more often than unilateral Hands, head, and neck; laryngeal Least apparent at rest; worsens with movement Aggravated by stress, fatigue, caffeine, and medications as above Improved by alcohol ingestion
Parkinson's tremor (pill-rolling tremor)	Resting tremor; does not worsen with movement (may actually improve) Varying amplitude, low frequency, "coarse" Asymmetrical Hands almost exclusively involved, legs rarely involved Unchanged with alcohol use

ual to sit with both hands and legs motionless in the chair while you observe for any tremor.

Bradykinesia

Bradykinesia (slowness of movement) may be recognized early as a paucity of facial muscle movements, causing what is termed a masked facies. The patient looks almost motionless in expression and lacks normal, eye-blinking frequency. The vocal quality of a parkinsonian patient is decreased (hypophonia), and his or her handwriting becomes slower and smaller (micrographia). As the larger muscles become involved, this condition is manifested as a slow, shuffling gait with a decreased arm swing. Bradykinesia is responsible for the loss of the normal fidgety movements of life, such as adjustments in sitting or standing positions, crossing or uncrossing the legs, or drumming the fingers.

Testing

A patient should be asked to rise from his or her chair and walk across the room. This allows the physician to observe the slowness and impreciseness of movements.

Rigidity

Rigidity (stiffness of movement) is the result of poor control of normal muscle activity. Fluid movements result from perfect contraction and relaxation of competitive muscles. In Parkinson's disease, the control of muscles is not precise, and paired agonist-antagonist muscles simultaneously contract, resulting in rigidity. Early in the disease, rigidity can best be appreciated in the wrist and elbow by active range of motion testing. Individual muscles have normal bulk and tone.

Testing

Test for rigidity by repetitive, passive range of motion of the upper extremity at both the elbow (flexion/extension) and the wrist (supination/pronation). The Parkinson's patient will have musculature resistance to this motion; coupled with tremor, such repetitive movements feel to the examiner "ratchety" or what is called "cogwheeling."

Other Characteristic Physical Findings

Seborrheic dermatitis is a scaly, mildly erythematous rash located in the scalp, eyebrows, and in the crevices around the nose and behind the ears. It is a very common rash in all age groups, but is particularly prevalent and severe in patients with Parkinson's disease. The pathophysiologic explanation for this association is not known.

Sialorrhea (excessive drooling) is common in patients with Parkinson's disease. This can result in chelitis, or skin breakdown, and maceration at the corners of the mouth. Sialorrhea is blamed on the lack of swallowing effort and frequency. Testing is by observation.

Postural instability (loss of balance) and *akinesia* (difficulty initiating movement) are commonly included with tremor, bradykinesia, and rigidity as cardinal features of Parkinson's disease. This feature is usually a later finding in the disease process and results from advancing bradykinesia and poor muscle control. Maintaining one's balance is a complex neurologic interaction of sensory and motor function. The perfect contraction and relaxation sequence permits one to stand and walk without teetering or falling. The patient with Parkinson's disease will have contracted flexor muscles greater than extensors and will stand stooped with flexion at the hips, knees, and trunk. As the patient's balance is challenged, he or she will have the tendency to lean backward (retropulsion) and be unable to have sufficient extensor control to maintain equilibrium. Gait observation (especially with turns) can reveal unsteadiness of position in space. Rhomberg testing (standing erect, arms at side, and eyes closed) will reveal any drifting from side to side and a propensity toward retropulsion.

Micrographia is a common way to deduce early Parkinson's disease. Also, the progression of the illness can be followed through evaluating for micrographia. A comparison of current and previous signatures or handwritten sentences will demonstrate a fine tremor to the lettering and a progressive reduction in handwriting size and flare, indicative of the disease.

Cognitive and affective changes are common in patients with Parkinson's disease. As in every geriatric patient, some type of mental status and depression screening should be included in the evaluation. The most commonly used screening tests are the Mini Mental Status Exam (see Appendix) and the Yesavage or Beck Depression Scales.

DIAGNOSTIC TEST DATA

Parkinson's disease is a clinical diagnosis without confirmatory laboratory or radiographic tests. The role of diagnostic testing is only to distinguish cases resulting from metabolic or structural lesions that damage the substantia nigra. Metabolic damage to these basal ganglion cells results from toxins such as carbon monoxide, cyanide, manganese, methylphenyltetrahydropyridine (MPTP) (a synthetic drug isolated in designer laboratories manufacturing meperidine), methanol, or mercury. Usually, some history of exposure or drug use is illicited in the medical history. Structural lesions such as basal ganglion tumors or arteriovenous malformations can be ruled out with computed tomography or magnetic resonance imaging. Such patients typically have signs or symptoms of sensory or motor losses.

DIFFERENTIAL DIAGNOSIS

There are two key issues in the differential diagnosis of patients with Parkinson's disease:

Does the Patient Have Parkinsonian Symptoms?

The clinical features of tremor, bradykinesia, and rigidity, when present in a constellation, define parkinsonism. Each feature alone or in some combination can be seen in patients who do not have parkinsonism. Tremor, bradykinesia, rigidity, balance disturbances, and miscellaneous findings should be demonstrated and distinguished from similar findings in other illnesses. Parkinsonian tremor needs to be distinguished from essential and physiologic tremors. Gait disorders such as those from strokes, tumors, musculoskeletal diseases, or other neurologic diseases must be clearly separated from the shuffling gait of Parkinson's disease. Rigidity and cogwheeling can be mimicked by muscular spasticity or paratonias. Miscellaneous features such as the masked facies, seborrhea, sialorrhea, and micrographia all can add certainty to the clinical diagnosis.

Are the Findings the Result of Idiopathic Parkinson's Disease or Something Else (Such as a Condition Secondary to an Identifiable Cause or Part of Another Neurodegenerative Syndrome)?

Eighty percent of all patients with parkinsonian symptoms have them as a result of idiopathic degeneration of the substantia nigra neurons, which is called Parkinson's disease. It has been referred to as primary parkinsonism and is different from secondary parkinsonism (parkinsonism from some secondary cause). There are a number of rarer neurodegenerative disorders that can have parkinsonian features but that also have other associated symptoms, which are occasionally referred to as Parkinson's plus syndromes. The differentiation between primary, secondary, and Parkinson's plus is important, because some of the secondary causes are reversible, and only primary Parkinson's disease reliably responds to levodopa therapy (Tables 7.2 and 7.3).

WHEN TO REFER

The family physician can confidently diagnose and treat patients with Parkinson's disease and other parkinsonian illnesses (particularly, medication-induced parkinsonism). If the diagnosis is in doubt, initial therapy is ineffective. Or there are atypical features, referral to a neurologist should be considered. Consideration should also be given to referring patients with Parkinson's plus syndromes.

MANAGEMENT

The treatment goals are to minimize symptoms and to prevent decline in function. Key issues in the management of the patient with Parkinson's disease include the following:

* Better control of the disease can be facilitated by establishing a consistent, predictable routine for the patient that reduces stress and encourages daily exercise.

TABLE 7.2. Causes of Secondary Parkinsonism

Medication induced
 Major tranquilizers (phenothiazines)
 Antihypertensives (reserpine [Serpasil], methyldopa [Aldomet])
 Dopamine antagonists (metochlopramide [Reglan], amoxapine [Asendin])
Encephalitis
Toxins
 Carbon monoxide, cyanide, manganese, methanol, MPTP
Head trauma

TABLE 7.3. Parkinsonian Findings in Association with Parkinson's Plus Syndromes

Multiple-system atrophy
  Shy-Drager
  Olivopontocerebellar degeneration
  Striatonigral degeneration
Progressive supranuclear palsy
  Paresis of vertical gaze, pseudobulbar palsy, postural instability, locomotion preserved
Dementia syndromes
  Alzheimer's disease
  Creutzfeldt–Jakob disease
Huntington's disease

- Every patient with Parkinson's disease should participate in ongoing, physical and occupational therapy, psychologic counseling, and support groups. Those with speech disturbances will benefit from speech therapy.
- In patients with medication-induced parkinsonism, the offending agent should be withdrawn. Symptoms will abate over a few days to months.
- The rate of clinical deterioration varies considerably among affected individuals. Patients with dementia generally have a more rapid progression and a worse prognosis.
- Most patients die with, not of, Parkinson's disease. However, the progressive immobility of some patients leads to life-threatening infections in both the respiratory system and in sites of skin breakdown.

Pharmacotherapy

Replacing the neurotransmitter dopamine, in the form of levodopa (Larodopa), is the basis of drug therapy for Parkinson's disease. Medications only treat the symptoms; no drug alters the disease process. In one study the drug selegiline (Eldepryl) was shown to slow the progression of the illness; however, the effect is limited, and follow-up studies have been unable to confirm this finding.

Medication side effects are neurologic, including the development of abnormal movements and mental status changes. The symptoms of Parkinson's disease fluctuate by the hour and by the day, so effectiveness of therapy should be judged on a long-term basis. The medications used have a narrow therapeutic window, and small changes can mean the difference in efficacy or the development of side effects.

Dopamine Enhancement

Levodopa is the most effective drug for the treatment of rigidity and bradykinesia in Parkinson's disease. It will also improve seborrhea, sialorrhea, and tremor, but less consistently than it ameliorates motor function. Levodopa crosses the blood-brain barrier and is converted to dopamine within the basal ganglion cells. The same enzymatic conversion, by dopa decarboxylase, occurs in the peripheral tissues, and the resulting dopamine cannot cross into the brain. Peripheral dopamine causes nausea, vomiting, and orthostatic hypotension.

Carbidopa (Lodosyn), a peripheral dopa-decarboxylase inhibitor, inhibits this conversion to dopamine outside the blood-brain barrier, reducing potential side effects. When given in combination with levodopa, it increases the amount of levodopa available in the brain. Therefore the combination of carbidopa/levodopa (Sinemet) is the standard formulation used in treating Parkinson's disease. Carbidopa/levodopa is best taken on an empty stomach to avoid competition with food for absorption.

Dosing.   Optimal dosing of carbidopa/levodopa depends on maximally inhibiting the peripheral dopa decarboxylase, which requires between 75 and 100 mg of carbidopa per day, with side effects occurring if more than 200 mg per day is used. The minimal, effective levodopa dose, when combined with the effective carbidopa dose, is 300 mg. Most patients will require 500 to 1000 mg per day. Tablets are available in 10/100-mg, 25/100-mg, and 25/250-mg (carbidopa/levodopa) formulations, with the usual starting dosage of either 25/100 mg or 25/250 mg, given three times a day. A long-acting combination of 50/200 mg is now available; however, its use is limited by both cost and the need for shorter-acting dosing for efficacy. "Wearing off" may occur at the end of the interdose interval after years of treatment. This can be somewhat alleviated by using smaller doses administered more frequently.

Side Effects.   Side effects of levodopa are frequent, disturbing, and limit its usefulness. Nausea, anorexia, flushing, hypotension, and cardiac arrhythmias are all peripheral side effects that are minimized by the correct dosing of carbidopa. The neurologic effects from levodopa include confusion, hallucinations, and bothersome movement disorders such as dyskinesias and akathisias. These two, movement-disorder side effects are characterized by abnormal excessive movements of the head, arms, trunk, and legs.

One of the most difficult problems with levodopa therapy is the marked fluctuation and diminution of its effectiveness over 3 to 5 years of use (the so-called "on/off" and "wearing off" phenomenon). The duration of action of a single dose also declines with time. All of these changes are ameliorated by increasing the dosage and frequency of levodopa, particularly the use of the 10/100-mg formulation of carbidopa/levodopa that can be given every 1 to 2 hours. Dietary protein is a particular problem and should be limited in patients taking levodopa.

All other medications and treatments should be considered only adjunctive. A description of the more commonly used adjuncts follows.

Dopamine Agonist Therapy

Bromocriptine (Parlodel) and pergolide (Permax), like levodopa, are useful for the rigidity and bradykinesia of Parkinson's disease. They also alleviate two bothersome symptoms that occasionally affect some patients—restless legs and painful dystonic cramps. Pramipexole (Mirapex) and ropinrole (Requip) are two new dopamine agonists approved for treatment of both early (without levodopa) and advanced (with levodopa) Parkinson's disease.

Mechanism of Action. The dopamine agonists act directly on the postsynaptic dopamine receptors to stimulate them as dopamine would. These drugs are usually not as effective as levodopa and are usually used alone only when levodopa side effects limit its use. Frequently, these drugs are combined with levodopa to reduce the need for higher and potentially more toxic doses. Their addition is often considered when "on/off" and "wearing off" effects occur.

Dosing. Bromocriptine is initiated at a low dose of 1.25 mg once or twice a day and titrated up over 2 to 3 weeks. Daily doses as high as 15 to 30 mg divided three times a day have been used. Pergolide is more potent on a mg/mg basis, and initial doses are 0.05 mg once a day, titrated up to 1 mg three times a day. The initial dosage of pramipexole is 0.125 mg twice daily, which can be doubled in the second week and again in the third week, and then to 0.75 mg twice daily in the fourth week. Increases of up to a maximum of 4.5 mg per day can be made weekly. Ropinirole is initially dosed at 0.25 mg three times daily and then can be increased by 0.25 mg per dose each week for the first 4 weeks. Patients who do not respond to one of these agents may respond to the other, as the drugs act on different dopamine receptors.

Side Effects. The side effects are similar to those of levodopa. All dopamine agonists can cause nausea and somnolence and can worsen dyskinesias. Syncope, occasionally associated with bradycardia or orthostatic hypotension, may occur. Finally, these medications are very expensive.

Anticholinergics

Anticholinergic medications are among the oldest drugs used to treat Parkinson's disease. These agents have only a minimal effect on the symptoms of rigidity and bradykinesia. They are most effective on tremor and sialorrhea. Doses should not exceed the middle range (100 mg twice daily for most common preparations) because of side effects. Benztropine (Cogentin) may also reduce symptoms in doses of 0.5 mg to 6 mg daily. Trihexyphenidyl (Artane) in doses of 2 to 5 mg three times daily may relieve tremor dramatically for a short period.

Mechanism of Action. The anticholinergics have the ability to decrease cholinergic activity, restore the balance of reduced dopamine to cholinergic neurotransmission. No one drug in this class is superior to another.

Side Effects. Unfortunately, these agents have a high-side-effect profile in elderly patients, including dry mouth, constipation, incontinence, and cognitive dysfunction, and therefore have only a minor role in treating Parkinson's disease.

Amantadine
Amantadine (Symmetrel) provides modest relief of tremor and some lessening of rigidity and bradykinesia.

Mechanism of Action. Amantadine is prescribed for influenza prophylaxis and during such use has been noted to improve some parkinsonian symptoms. However, amantadine is a minor drug in the armamentarium for treating Parkinson's disease. It can be used as a single agent early in the disease or in combination with carbidopa/levodopa to smooth out patients' symptoms.

Dosing. The usual dosing is 100 to 300 mg per day.

Side Effects. Confusion, edema, and livedo reticularis may occur.

Neuroprotector Therapy
Selegiline is a monoamine oxidase β-receptor inhibitor. In one study, selegiline was shown to delay the need for carbidopa/levodopa therapy when used early in Parkinson's disease, which led to its being touted as the only drug available that prevented the progression of Parkinson's disease. However, subsequent studies with this drug have not been as convincing, and a question of increased mortality in patients using carbidopa/levodopa concomitantly has been raised. Another factor limiting its use is the virtual lack of symptom improvement in patients treated with selegiline. It has little effect on tremor, rigidity, or bradykinesia. At this point, it is unclear what role selegiline has in the treatment of Parkinson's disease.

Antidepressants
Depression is a common accompaniment of Parkinson's disease, seen in up to 40% of patients in some studies. Antidepressants are the mainstay of therapy, with selective serotonin reuptake inhibitors (SSRIs) being prescribed most frequently because of their low-side-effect profile. However, selegiline and SSRIs used in combination can cause a serotonin syndrome, characterized by delusional behavior, tachycardia, hypertension, diaphoresis, and, occasionally, death. Also, selegiline and monoamine oxidase inhibitors (MAOI) are contraindicated. (See Chapter 4 for a discussion of antidepressant medications.)

Surgery

Surgery may be indicated for patients for whom levodopa treatment has lost its efficacy and who are disabled by motor dysfunction caused by inability to use medication or the use of excessive medication. Three surgical procedures have been used to alleviate symptoms in patients with Parkinson's disease. Two procedures are ablative, destroying the thalamus or the globus pallidum. Thalamotomy and pallidotomy are both stereotactic procedures that are used in younger patients with refractory bradykinesias and rigidity. Dysarthria has been reported as a common complication of bilateral thalamotomy. Other complications of surgical procedures include infarction, hemiparesis, and/or confusion. Unilateral thalamotomy appears promising with a beneficial effect on rigidity and dyskinesias. The third surgical procedure available to treat Parkinson's patients is fetal dopaminergic cell transplantation, which is experimental at this time.

FOLLOW-UP

Management focuses on symptom control and skillful use of potentially toxic medications. Levodopa, and the other adjuvant therapies, all have to be carefully monitored for their side effects. Management focuses on symptom control and skillful use of potentially toxic medications. Levodopa, and the other adjuvant therapies, all have to be carefully monitored for their side effects.

Symptom control underlies the key issue of function. A functional assessment, including activities of daily living, instrumental activities of daily living, and cognitive and affective function, are important components to follow-up visits. Since symptoms are the key to drug doses and choices, careful assessment of the patient is the most important factor. For patients who are dependent on caregiver support, an evaluation of the stress on the caregiver is also important.

Early in Parkinson's disease, patients can be followed with one or two visits a year. As the disease progresses, visits will increase to monthly. Since each medication used to treat this disease has a narrow therapeutic window, the key to successful therapy is a balance of symptom control and adverse drug effects. The natural history of the disease is to have variations in symptoms on a daily or even hourly basis. Symptom control requires appropriate drug doses given at appropriate times. Medication doses and types may need to be increased or decreased or given more or less frequently depending on symptoms.

Patients with Parkinson's disease will have a slowly progressive course, characterized by worsening symptoms. Patient and family education is the backbone of the primary care of these patients and their families.

PATIENT EDUCATION

As a neurodegenerative disorder, Parkinson's disease will inevitably progress. No therapies to date can stop the ongoing destruction of dopaminergic cells and the development of worsening symptoms. Patients and families need to fully understand the disease and its management and to participate in assessing the effects and toxicities of medication.

TABLE 7.4. Resources for Patients

American Parkinson's Disease Association, Inc.
1250 Hylan Blvd., Suite 4B
Staten Island, NY 10305
800-223-2732

National Parkinson's Foundation
1501 N.W. 9th Ave. Bob Hope Road
Miami, Florida 33136-1494
800-327-4545

Parkinson's Disease Foundation
710 West 168th Street
New York, N.Y. 10032
800-457-6676

Early in the course of the disease, the patient will lead a normal life. He or she can eat a regular diet, although low protein and high roughage is recommended to improve the absorption of levodopa and to increase water content of the stool to avoid constipation. Patients with early Parkinson's can continue to work and drive.

Symptoms are generally controllable for a number of years. Unfortunately, the disease will progress and the symptoms will become harder to control. As the disease progresses, disability makes working and driving impossible.

Changes in diet (especially protein intake) or activity level or use of over-the-counter medications with anticholinergic or antihistamine effects can significantly worsen symptoms.

Patients may gain more information from the organizations listed in Table 7.4. A patient information sheet is included in the Appendix.

SUGGESTED READINGS

Calne DB. Treatment of Parkinson's disease. N Engl J Med 1993;329:1021–1027.

Calne DB, Snow BJ, Lel C, et al. Criteria for diagnosing Parkinson's disease. Ann Neurol 1992;32:S125–127.

Hely MA, Morris JG. Controversies in the treatment of Parkinson's disease. Curr Opin Neurol 1996;9:308–313.

Koller WC, Huber SJ. Tremor disorders of aging: diagnosis and management. Geriatrics 1989;44:33–36.

Manyam BV. Practical guidelines for management of Parkinson disease. J Am Board Fam Pract 1997;10:412–424.

Marsden CD. Neurological management: Parkinson's disease. J Neurol Neurosurg Psychiatr 1994;57:672–681.

CHAPTER 8

Urinary Incontinence

Urinary incontinence is the uncontrollable, unanticipated loss of urine causing wetting of clothes and body. Incontinence occurs in up to 35% of all persons over 60 years of age and in up to 50% of elderly patients in hospitals. Women have twice the incidence of men. It is useful to classify incontinence in the following way:

- Temporary incontinence—caused by an easily reversible medical condition (30 to 50% of all cases)
- Fixed incontinence—symptoms are more chronic (50 to 70% of all cases); best thought of in four categories:
  - Urge—spontaneous uncontrolled emptying of the bladder
  - Stress—involuntary loss of small amount of urine secondary to increased intraabdominal pressure
  - Overflow—leakage of small amounts of urine from a distended bladder
  - Functional—inability to use toilet facilities for a reason not directly related to the genitourinary tract

CHIEF COMPLAINT

Patients with urinary incontinence frequently will not discuss symptoms with their physician. The social stigma and embarrassment associated with incontinence cause many to live with the condition rather than seek treatment. As part of their routine history and physical examination, all elderly patients should be asked about loss of urine. The following questions have been recommended in the Agency for Health Care Policy and Research Clinical Practice Guidelines on Urinary Incontinence.

- Do you ever lose urine when you don't want to?
- Do you ever wear a protective pad to catch urine?
- Do you ever lose urine when you cough, sneeze, or laugh?

HISTORY

A detailed history will lead to the most likely diagnosis. First, determine whether the incontinence is a short-term or long-term problem. Short-term, or transient urinary incontinence, is frequently caused by easily diagnosed and treatable conditions. Long-term causes of urinary incontinence are best thought of in four categories: stress, urge, overflow, and functional (Table 8.1).

The historical findings will help determine into which category the urinary incontinence falls.

Key questions to ask include the following:

- Does the incontinence occur with sneezing, coughing, or laughing? (stress)
- Does the incontinence occur with symptoms of an urgency to void? (urge)
- What is the volume of urine lost? Large amounts? (urge) Small amounts? (stress; overflow)
- Do you have symptoms of voiding difficulty such as hesitancy, dribbling, or nocturia associated with the incontinence? (overflow)

TABLE 8.1. Classification of Persistent Urinary Incontinence

Type	Symptoms	Physical Findings	Possible Cause
Stress	Small volume of urine loss associated with increased intra-abdominal pressure (such as that occurring during a cough, sneeze or upon standing)	Loss of urine with cough or Valsalva maneuver; perhaps cystocele	Laxity of pelvic floor musculature
Urge	Large volume of urine loss associated with urgency to void	None	Abnormal contraction of bladder muscle, also known as premature vesicular contraction
Overflow	Small volume urine loss with distended bladder	Enlarged bladder with obstruction or urethra or atonic bladder; large prostate or pelvic mass	Atonic bladder caused by diabetes, spinal cord injury; obstructed bladder, caused by large prostate or pelvic mass tumor
Functional	Mixed volume loss associated with nonbladder/nonurinary system disease	Dementia or physical limitation/restriction such as severe osteoarthritis or rheumatoid arthritis, end-stage Parkinson's disease, or physical restraint	Intact urinary system; incontinence secondary to disease (other than that of genitourinary system)

- Do you have difficulty finding the bathroom or using the toilet once you have found the bathroom? (functional)

Additional useful information includes the following:

- The patient's most bothersome symptom
- Other urinary tract symptoms (nocturia, hesitancy, etc.)
- Daily fluid intake
- Bowel habits
- Changes in sexual function and habits
- Prior treatments
- Environmental assessment
- Social and daily activities
- Treatment expectations

A commonly used historical aid is to ask the patient or the family/caregiver to keep a "voiding diary" for 1 to 2 weeks. This diary should include details of continent, as well as incontinent, voiding episodes, their time and volume, as well as any associated factors, and fluid intake. With this information, the clinician can get a clearer picture of the patient's urinary and hydration habits.

PHYSICAL EXAMINATION

The physical examination can reveal key factors in patients with urinary incontinence. The following areas should be carefully assessed:

- Overall fluid status
- Abdominal examination
- Vascular and neurologic function
- Findings of potential endocrinologic diseases (diabetic retinopathy, skin changes, and cataracts; hyperthyroid tremor, goiter, and hypothyroid skin changes and diminished reflexes; truncal obesity, oily skin and acne, easy bruising, and "buffalo" hump associated with cortisol disorder)
- Urogenital exam. In men, the rectal exam can determine prostate size and contour, as well as presence or absence of masses. Rectal tone, perineal sensation, and cremasteric reflex are good indicators of the status of the neurologic system.
- Pelvic exam. In women, the pelvic exam reveals many important factors. The patient's hormonal status is important and can be determined by careful inspection of the vaginal walls. Lack of estrogen creates dry, thin, friable vaginal mucosa and can alter the periurethral tissue, leading to urinary incontinence. Pelvic or rectal masses are important to identify. The presence of uterine prolapse and/or a cystocele is important to document.

- Direct observation of urine loss (full bladder using cough stress test)
- Mental status exam
- Functional exam

DIAGNOSTIC TEST DATA

Office Maneuvers

1. The "pad test" is an easy office test to determine the competency of the uretheral sphincter in women. The test is performed as follows:
   - The female patient is asked to stand.
   - The physician places a dry absorbent pad between the patient's legs.
   - The patient is asked to cough or perform the Valsalva maneuver.
   - Any leakage of urine onto the pad indicates the presence of stress incontinence.
2. The "post-void residual test" is a relatively simple way to determine contractile function of the bladder. It is useful in both men and women to determine bladder atony or obstruction.
   - The patient is asked to void completely and then to return to the office exam room.
   - The bladder is catheterized, and the amount of urine left in the bladder is determined.

Post-void residual of less than 100 mL is normal; over 200 mL is abnormal. An equivocal finding is 100 to 200 mL. Patients with abnormal post-void residuals should be considered for urologic referral for cystoscopy and cystometrogram.

Laboratory Testing

The most important laboratory test is the urinalysis (Table 8.2). Potential underlying etiologies may be indicated by abnormal findings such as the following:

- Pyuria
- Hematuria
- Heavy proteinuria

TABLE 8.2. Possible Interpretation of Abnormal Urinary Findings in Patients with Incontinence

Finding	Possible Interpretation
Pyuria	Urinary tract infection
Hematuria	Malignancy, infection, kidney stone
Proteinuria	Renal disease, diabetes mellitus

TABLE 8.3. Laboratory Screening Tests to Determine Cause of Urinary Incontinence

Blood test	Disease
Serum electrolytes, serum osmolarity, urine osmolarity	Diabetes insipidus
TSH, thyroid panel	Thyroid disease
Serum cortisol, dexamethasone suppression test	Adrenocortical disorder
Prostate-specific antigen	Prostate cancer
Decreased blood urea nitrogen, increased mean corpuscular volume	Alcoholism

Other laboratory tests have a low yield, but should be done when clinical suspicion exists (Table 8.3). Screening blood tests can be done for occult diabetes, prostate cancer, other causes of transient urinary incontinence.

Cystoscopy and cystometrograms are not necessary in the routine treatment of urinary incontinence.

DIFFERENTIAL DIAGNOSIS

The differential diagnosis of urinary incontinence is divided initially into two categories:

- Transient urinary incontinence (duration of less than 1 month)
- Persistent urinary incontinence

Transient Urinary Incontinence

The underlying causes of urinary incontinence of acute onset/short duration can be remembered using the mnemonic DIAPPERS.

D = Delirium
I = Infections
A = Atrophic urethritis/vaginitis
P = Pharmaceuticals
P = Psychologic
E = Endocrine disorder/excessive urine production
R = Restricted mobility, urinary retention
S = Stool (fecal impaction)

Delirium

Patients with acute confusional states that persist for a sufficient duration will have urinary incontinence as a result of their mental status and the lack of sufficient cognitive function to remember to hold the urine. The incontinence is transient and will resolve when the confusional state resolves.

Infections

Urinary tract infection is one of the most common causes of transient urinary incontinence. When the infection is treated, the urinary incontinence will resolve. Asymptomatic bacteriuria, which is common in older adults, *does not* cause urinary incontinence. Fatigue and lethargy, symptoms of a systemic infection, can lead to urinary incontinence because they compromise a person's ability to get to the restroom in a timely manner. Also, systemic infection may result in a change in mental status.

Atrophic Urethritis/Vaginitis

In older women who are not receiving sufficient estrogen replacement, atrophic changes can occur in the vaginal and periurethral tissue that predispose the patient to urinary incontinence. With estrogen therapy, the urinary incontinence will resolve.

Pharmaceuticals

A variety of medications can cause urinary incontinence in the elderly:

- Sedatives and hypnotics such as benzodiazepines or alcohol can contribute to transient urinary incontinence by clouding the sensorium, impairing mobility, and inducing diuresis.
- Diuretics, or any medication that increases urinary flow, can cause a previously continent patient to become incontinent. Thiazide and the loop diuretics, as well as caffeine and alcohol, may cause the bladder to become overfull, leading to premature contraction.
- Anticholinergics, and drugs with anticholinergic properties, including many over-the-counter drugs, can cause relaxation of the bladder detrusor muscle, which has cholinergic receptors, and overdistention and/or urinary retention may result.
- α-Adrenergic agents can affect sphincter control in the proximal urethra, as it has α-receptors and is under adrenergic control.
- α-Agonists, including ephedrine and its derivatives, cause sphincter tightening. These drugs are found in many over-the-counter multicomponent cold remedies and can cause urinary retention and overflow incontinence.
- α-Antagonists, including some antihypertensives, cause relaxation of the urethral sphincter, and can cause urinary loss.
- Calcium-channel blockers affect the smooth bladder detrusor. Detrusor inactivity can lead to urinary retention and overflow incontinence.

Psychologic Conditions

Severe depression may occasionally be the underlying cause of urinary incontinence. Although the urinary incontinence is not purely transient, it will resolve if the underlying affective disorder is treated.

Endocrine Disorder/Excessive Urine Production

Transient urinary incontinence, secondary to both an increase in urine production and mental status changes, is often associated with the following metabolic disorders:

- Hyperglycemia
- Hypercalcemia
- Diabetes insipidus

Excessive urine production can also occur in the following settings:

- Congestive heart failure
- Polydipsia
- Edema caused by hypoalbuminemia

Restricted Mobility

Elderly persons with any degree of urgency for urination will display transient urinary incontinence if their mobility is restricted in any way. The classic scenario is a hospitalized elder who becomes incontinent because of the lack of timely response to the need for assistance with urination. A urinal or bedside commode will alleviate this problem. Osteoarthritis, Parkinson's disease, or others that limit mobility also play a role in urinary incontinence.

Stool (Fecal Impaction)

A fecal impaction will obstruct urinary flow and result in urinary retention or cause bladder irritation and a premature contraction. Disimpaction will restore continence.

Persistent Urinary Incontinence

Persistent urinary incontinence can be classified into the following four groups by underlying pathophysiology.

Stress Incontinence

Stress incontinence is defined as an involuntary loss of small amounts of urine secondary to increased intraabdominal pressure, such as occurs with coughing, sneezing, changing to an upright posture, or exercising, that overcomes a weak urinary sphincter. The underlying pathophysiology is weakness or laxity of the pelvic floor musculature and/or the urethral sphincter. It occurs almost exclusively in women; the typical patient is multiparous and has an associated cystocele or uterine prolapse.

Atrophic vaginal changes and the use of α-adrenergic blocking agents are associated with a transient form of this type of urinary incontinence. It can also occur in men with a history of urethral trauma.

Urge Incontinence

Urge incontinence is defined as the spontaneous, uncontrolled emptying of the bladder. It occurs equally in men and women. The sense of urgency to void is accompanied by premature vesicular contractions that increase the bladder pressure sufficiently to overcome urethral resistance and cause leakage of large volumes of urine.

The key to understanding urge incontinence is discovering why the bladder contracts at an inappropriate time. Premature vesicular contractions may be caused by the following:

- Neurologic disease at a local or central nervous system level (referred to as "detrusor hyperreflexia")
- Local conditions, such as cystitis, bladder tumor, urinary stones, or bladder diverticuli uretheritis, that irritate the detrusor muscle, causing it to dysfunction (referred to as "detrusor instability or irritability")
- Detrusor irritability, which may also arise from problems with the smooth muscle itself

Overflow Incontinence

Overflow incontinence is defined as the leakage of small amounts of urine from an overdistended bladder and can occur as a result of the following:

- Anatomic obstruction to outflow, such as a large prostate, uterine or cervical pathology, uretheral strictures, bladder neck tumors, or extrinsic compression from fecal impaction
- Use of an α-agonist or anticholinergic agent
- A hypotonic and overdistended bladder resulting from lack of detrusor muscle function caused by intrinsic bladder muscle disease; overdistention occurs more commonly in men than in women
- Atonic bladder resulting from lack of neurologic input (spinal cord injury, diabetes, etc.)

The diagnosis of overflow incontinence is made by a history of small-volume urine loss and the finding of an overdistended bladder or bladder with a large post-void residual.

Functional Urinary Incontinence

Functional urinary incontinence is defined as urinary loss associated with the inability to use toileting facilities secondary to cognitive, physical, or emotional disorders and is not directly related to genitourinary pathology. Volume of urine loss is variable, depending on the bladder capacity at the time of a void, but is usually moderate to large as opposed to dribbling. Patient has no discernible pathology, but seems unable or unwilling to maintain continence. This type of incontinence commonly occurs in patients with moderate to severe dementia.

Mixed Urinary Incontinence

The etiology of urinary incontinence is often multifactorial:

• Stress and urge incontinence commonly occurs in older women.
• Urge and overflow incontinence occurs often in frail, nursing-home patients.
• Functional incontinence occurs in combination with other forms of incontinence in persons with dementia.
• Patients with persistent urinary incontinence can have episodes of urine loss that are caused by one of the transient mechanisms.

WHEN TO REFER

The family physician plays a key role in the diagnosis and management of urinary incontinence. Referral for more-advanced workup or consultation should be considered if any of the following occur:

• The diagnosis or choice of appropriate therapy is unclear.
• The post-void residual is abnormal (>200 mL).
• There is evidence of an underlying malignancy such as hematuria or a palpable mass.
• Therapy has been unsuccessful.

MANAGEMENT

Figure 8.1 is an algorithm for evaluation and managment of urinary incontinence. Treatment options for patients with urinary incontinence fall into five categories:

• Treatment of underlying conditions, if present
• Behavioral intervention
• Medications
• Surgery
• Protection from ongoing urinary incontinence (catheterization, pads, etc.)

Treatment of Underlying Condition

Transient incontinence can often be ameliorated or resolved by management of the underlying condition and removal of risk factors (Table 8.4).

Behavioral Intervention

Voiding Diary

A voiding diary is a useful tool for patients with any type of urinary incontinence. Patients are asked to document continent and incontinent voids for 1 week. The following should be detailed:

TABLE 8.4. Treatable Causes of Urinary Incontinence

Cerebrovascular accident
Decreased mobility
Diabetes
Diminished cognitive status and delirium
Environmental barriers
Estrogen depletion
Fecal impaction
High-impact physical activities
High fluid intake
Offending medications
Pelvic muscle weakness

- Timing
- An estimate of volume of urine voided or lost
- The surrounding situation

Toileting Programs

A schedule of timed voidings is the simplest, most successful, and therefore most widely used behavioral intervention. The patient voids on a schedule rather than on an as-needed basis. The voiding frequency may be as often as every 30 minutes for some patients, but can usually be stretched to every 2 to 3 hours. This can be accomplished by the patient if he or she is cognitively and physically capable, or with assistance from a caregiver. Maintaining a low bladder volume by following a voiding schedule will decrease all forms of urinary incontinence and can alleviate the need for indwelling catheters or diapers.

In cognitively impaired patients, a stimulus such as lower abdominal pressure, stroking the inner thigh, or running water may be required.

Pelvic Floor Exercises

Kegel exercises have been documented to benefit patients with stress urinary incontinence and are easy to teach. A set of patient instructions are located in the Appendix.

Vaginal Weight Training

This technique can be used to increase periurethral muscle strength by exercising pelvic muscles.

Electrical Stimulation

Electrical stimulation to afferent fibers through an intravaginal electrode inhibits bladder instability and improves contractility and efficiency. This technique requires specialized training.

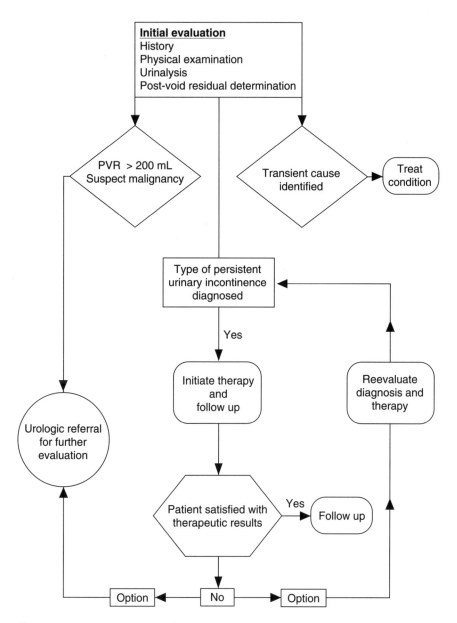

FIGURE 8.1. Algorithm for evaluation and management of urinary incontinence. *PVR,* postvoid residual.

Biofeedback

Although it has been shown to be effective, it may not be a practical behavioral option. With this technique, biofeedback equipment is used to help the patient recognize the physiologic response associated with both the need to void and the activity of voiding. However, the usefulness of this approach is limited by unavailability and low patient acceptance.

Pharmacologic Agents

Refer to Table 8.5 for information about specific medications.

Stress Urinary Incontinence

Drug therapy is directed at (1) treating atrophic changes in the perineal tissue and (2) strengthening the sphincter tone of the urethra. Frequently, patients are prescribed agents directed at both objectives at once.

Estrogens are the mainstay of treatment for atrophic vaginitis/urethritis; they can be given topically or orally. Topical estrogen improves symptoms more rapidly than oral formulations; however, patients usually prefer the oral estrogens. It is common to prescribe both oral and topical therapy and to discontinue the topical applications after 3 to 4 weeks of combined use. Transdermal estrogens have not been studied in the treatment of urinary incontinence, but can probably be substituted for oral estrogens.

Sympathetic α-receptor agonists will cause contraction of the smooth muscle around the urethra, leading to tightening of the urethral sphincter. Some commonly used α-agonists include the following:

- Phenylpropanolamine (Ornade)
- Pseudoephedrine (Sudafed)
- Imipramine (Tofranil)

Urge Urinary Incontinence

Medications that inhibit contractions of the detrusor muscle, a smooth muscle, include the following:

- Probantheline (Pro-Banthine), an anticholinergic
- Oxybutynin (Ditropan), a smooth-muscle relaxant with anticholinergic properties
- Calcium-channel blockers
- Imipramine, an anticholinergic and α-adrenergic

Overflow Urinary Incontinence

Overflow urinary incontinence is commonly resistant to pharmacologic therapy. Cholinergic agents that stimulate bladder contraction such as bethanechol (Urecholine) are rarely able to restore continence.

α-Adrenergic blockers such as terazosin (Hytrin) may decrease urinary ob-

TABLE 8.5.   Pharmacologic Treatment of Urinary Incontinence

Drug Class	Specific Medications and Dosages	Mechanism of Action	Type of Incontinence	Adverse Effects
Conjugated estrogens	Oral: 0.625 mg QD Topical: 0.5 to 1 g three to four times per week	Strengthens perineal tissue	Stress	Endometrial cancer (must add progestin with prolonged use)
α-Adrenergic agonists	Pseudoephedrine (Sudafed)[a], 15 to 30 mg three times daily; Phenylpropanolamine (Entex, Ornade, Contact)[a], 25 mg q 4–6 hours or 75 mg q 12 hours; Imipramine (Tofranil)[a], 10 to 50 mg three times daily	Increases urethral smooth-muscle contraction and urethral sphincter tone	Stress	Headache, tachycardia, increases blood pressure
Anticholinergic and/or anti-spasmodic agents	Oxybutynin (Ditropan), 2.5 to 5 mg three times daily; Probantheline (Pro-Banthine), 15 to 30 mg three times daily; Imipramine[a], 10 to 50 mg three times daily	Diminishes involuntary bladder contractions	Urge	Dry mouth, blurry vision, confusion, urinary retention
Cholinergic agents	Bethanechol (Urecholine), 10 to 30 mg three times daily	Stimulates bladder contractions	Overflow	Bradycardia, hypotension, bronchospasm
α-Adrenergic antagonists	Terazosin (Hytrin), 1 to 10 mg daily	Relaxes urethral sphincter	Overflow	Hypotension

[a]These drugs are not approved by the U.S. Food and Drug Administration for use in urinary incontinence.

struction and allow for freer urinary flow; however, by the time incontinence develops, the obstruction may be too severe to be treated with medications.

Surgical Intervention

In some cases of urinary incontinence, particularly in stress incontinence, surgery can be effective. Surgery usually involves elevation of the bladder neck; it may include repair of cystocele, rectocele, or both and may also include uterine suspension or hysterectomy.

- For stress urinary incontinence, surgery should be considered after 3 to 6 months of nonsurgical therapy has failed. Surgery can include retropubic

suspension, sling (mostly in women) artificial sphincter placement, or ure-thral bulking.
- For urge urinary incontinence, surgery can include augmentation cysto-plasty.
- For overflow urinary incontinence secondary to obstruction, removal of the obstruction, usually an enlarged prostate or intraurethral mass or stric-ture, can result in return to continence.

Protection from Ongoing Urinary Incontinence
For a limited number of patients with urinary incontinence, catheterization is the only therapeutic option that is effective. There are three approaches to urethral catheterization: intermittent, chronic indwelling, and suprapubic.

Intermittent catheterization can be performed by a caregiver or by the pa-tient. Patients with spinal cord injuries or with an atonic bladder that does not respond to other therapies are the usual candidates for intermittent catheterization.

Intermittent catheterization is typically performed with a nonsterile, "clean" technique or, in immune-compromised, frail elders, with a sterile technique. The incidence of urinary infections with a clean, intermittent catheterization is lower than that among patients with chronic, indwelling catheters. There is good evidence that the use of prophylactic antibiotics to decrease the incidence of urinary infections in patients utilizing intermittent catheterization is not effective and only increases the likelihood of resistant organisms.

Chronic, indwelling catheterization may be the best choice in the follow-ing patients:

- Those who are terminally ill
- Those with perineal pressure ulcers
- Those who lack adequate caregiver support

Chronic, indwelling catheterization is often used in situations in which less invasive therapy would be effective, particularly in a nursing-home setting with functionally impaired patients. Published data show that 50% of nursing-home patients are incontinent and that the use of chronic indwelling catheterization is between 6 and 28 percent; the actual requirement for such use may be as low as 2 to 3%. Timed voidings combined with or without med-ication may be successful in eliminating or reducing the need for a chronic, indwelling catheter.

The risk of long-term, chronic, indwelling catheterization is significant. Bacteriuria is present in 100% of patients within 2 weeks of catheter place-ment. The rate of sepsis in nursing-home patients with an indwelling catheter is three times that of patients without catheters. The mortality rate among septic patients is also higher. Chronic, indwelling catheterization should be used only as a last resort. Other possible complications may include the following:

- Increased risk of renal damage
- Stone formation
- Trauma to the urethra and bladder
- Epididymitis and prostatitis
- Increased pain from bladder spasms

Key points to keep in mind in the use of a chronic, indwelling catheter include the following:

- For patients with a sterile, closed system, the catheter should be changed every 30 days unless encrustation creates blockage on a more frequent basis.
- There is no role for prophylactic antibiotics in patients with an indwelling catheter. If an infection develops, as judged by local or systemic symptoms, the following apply:
  - The old catheter should be removed and disposed of.
  - A new one should be inserted.
  - A urine specimen obtained from the new catheter should be sent for culture.

External compression devices are another option. In women with stress incontinence, devices that are self-adhesive to the perineum and obstruct the uretheral orifice are available without prescription at pharmacies. Although there have been no controlled studies involving these devices, and although their role in increasing the frequency of urinary tract infections is unclear, external compression devices may be considered as a temporary aid or may be used in patients for whom medication and surgery are not plausible.

FOLLOW-UP

Patients with urinary incontinence require periodic follow-up to evaluate continued efficacy of therapy and the possible development of recurrent urinary incontinence secondary to a transient or persistent cause.

PATIENT EDUCATION

A patient information sheet on urinary incontinence is included in the Appendix. The following are key points to convey to patients:

- Urinary incontinence is not a part of the normal aging process.
- Urinary incontinence is a sign of an underlying problem that might be treatable.

TABLE 8.6. Resources for Patients

National Institute on Aging Information Center
P.O. Box 8057
Gaithersburg, MD 20898-8057
800-222-2225

The NIA produces free-of-charge "Age Pages" on a number of topics; the one on urinary incontinence is excellent.

Alliance for Aging Research
2021 K Street, NW, Suite 305
Washington, DC 20006
800-293-2856
This group publishes patient-oriented information on a variety of topics.

- Bladder training and medications are the major treatment options.
- A diary of urinary and fluid-intake habits is very helpful to determine the cause of incontinence.
- Estrogen therapy is helpful in certain types of bladder-control problems.
- Because there are several causes of incontinence, medications should be started only after discussion with your family physician.
- Caffeine and alcohol intake may worsen bladder control problems.
- Resources (Table 8.6) are available to learn more about urinary incontinence.

SUGGESTED READINGS

AHCPR Guideline Update Panel. Urinary incontinence guidelines in adults. Managing acute and chronic urinary incontinence. Am Fam Phys 1996;54:5.

Mold JW. Pharmacotherapy of urinary incontinence. Am Fam Phys 1996;54:673–680.

Ouslander JG. Geriatric urinary incontinence. Dis Mon 1992;38:65–149.

Resnick NM, JG Ouslander. NIH Conference on urinary incontinence. J Am Geriatr Soc 1990;38:263–386.

Wells TJ, Brink CA, Diokno AC, et al. Pelvic muscle exercise for stress urinary incontinence in elderly women. J Am Geriatr Soc 1991;39:785–791.

CHAPTER 9

....

Falls

The incidence of falls increases with age, but will vary depending on the population studied. In community-dwelling healthy elders, one out of three is estimated to experience a fall in a year. Most of these falls are seen as "trips" or "minor falls" and are blamed on a number of factors by the patient. Many of these lesser events are not reported to the physician. In fact, only 5% of all falls result in a fracture. The rate of falls among nursing-home residents is close to 60% annually; the fracture rate is also higher at 25%. Annually, 1800 falls result in death.

Most falls in the elderly are multifactorial in cause and require a careful and thorough evaluation and management plan. The slowing of nerve conduction and the decline in proprioception affect the sense of balance and position, and have a dramatic effect on gait. Gait changes from that with a fluid arm swing, a narrow base, and a wide free step that can accommodate many uneven surfaces and missteps to a gait that is less free and more shuffling. A senior cannot afford a misstep, and the shortening of the arm swing, the narrowing of the step width, the widening of the base, and the slowing of the pace are attempts to ensure stability. These normal, age-related changes are frequently combined with pathologic changes such as arthritis, diabetic neuropathies, poor vision, and others, which result in a high incidence of falls. Patients who fall and sustain little injury often do not report it, so the physician should ask about falls as part of a routine exam in all elders.

To prevent morbidity and mortality it is our hope to detect risk factors early and to develop strategies to treat the underlying disorders. The changes in our physical abilities with aging are a major factor in the risk of falling.

Risk factors for falls are commonly broken into two categories (Table 9.1):

- Those that pertain to the person's physical status (intrinsic factors)
- Those that are related to the surrounding environment (extrinsic factors)

Although a single fall could result from one single cause such as an acute stroke or slipping on a wet surface, the majority of falls result from a combination of both intrinsic and extrinsic risk factors.

TABLE 9.1. Causes of Falls

Physical Status (Intrinsic)	Environmental Factors (Extrinsic)
Acute illnesses	Cracked or uneven pavement
Age >75 years	Lack of adequate railings or grab bars
Alcohol excesses	Poor lighting
Amputations	Slip rugs; unsecured carpeting or flooring
Cognitive dysfunction	Uneven stairs
Degenerative arthritis	Unstable furniture or low-lying pieces
Diseases causing nocturia	Wet or otherwise slippery surfaces
Diseases or deformities of the feet	Poor footwear
Dizziness	
Hip fractures	
Impaired vision and hearing	
Parkinson's disease	
Peripheral neuropathies	
Postural hypotension	
Previous lower extremity fractures	
Sedative–hypnotic medications	
Strokes with residual deficits	

CHIEF COMPLAINT

Falls are usually incidents reported by the patient or his or her family or friends. In many situations, patients will minimize the event or blame it on some external factor. In some situations the patient will not complain of any falling incidents, but will remember such episodes when asked directly. A useful question is "Have you fallen or tripped to an extent that you ended up on the ground?"

HISTORY

The specific detailed history of falls may need to be obtained from both the patient and any witnesses who can be found. This is a key factor in determining the falling risk factors and should not be overlooked. Questions should include the following:

- Where did the fall, or falls, occur?
- What was the condition of the environment?
- Was the fall inside or outside?
- Was there any furniture that caused the fall or grab bars that helped to prevent the fall?

- Were there stairs involved, and what was their condition, including railings and lighting?
- Was a rug or carpeting involved, or was the flooring uneven, wet, or slippery?
- What was the lighting?
- Were there any associated symptoms?
  - Premonitory?
  - Palpitations?
  - Chest pains?
  - Focal neurologic changes?
  - Loss of consciousness?
  - Incontinence?
  - Dyspnea?
  - Dizziness or lightheadedness?
  - Vertigo?
- What was the person wearing—specifically the type of footwear?
- Was he or she using any assistive devices such as canes, walkers, or visual or hearing aids? Is the device in good condition?
- Has the patient fallen before?

Other key points to cover during the history include the following:

- Underlying illnesses
- Past medical history
- Current prescription and over-the-counter medications. (Sedative hypnotics, antidepressants, anticholinergics, and alcohol are the leading drug groups associated with falls.)

PHYSICAL EXAMINATION

As falls are frequently the result of increasing frailty in the individual, it is important to evaluate the patient thoroughly (Table 9.2).The physical exam begins with an overall assessment of the patient's general medical condition, with particular attention to findings associated with the historical clues. Special attention should be given to examination of the following:

- Vital signs—These include pulse irregularities, blood pressure, temperature elevation, increased respiratory rate, and orthostatic hypotension.
- Musculoskeletal system—Evaluation of the musculoskeletal system should include both unilateral and bilateral findings. Motion at the hip, knee, and ankle are all essential for postural stability, and changes in these joints or their surrounding muscle strength can increase the risk of falling.
- Neurologic system—Changes in the neurologic system, both with aging and secondary to pathology, can increase the risk of falling. Motor and sensory function and reflexes should be evaluated.

TABLE 9.2. Essential Components of the Physical Examination

Vital signs
Mental status testing
Cardiac
Musculoskeletal
   Neurologic
   Proprioception
Vision
Hearing
Gait and balance testing

Reprinted with permission from Steinweg KK. The changing approach to falls in the elderly. Am Fam Physician 1997;56:1815–1822.

- Gait and balance—Assessment is critical in the evaluation and can identify more remedial causes of falls than the general neurologic or musculoskeletal exams.

There are a series of standardized assessment protocols for evaluating a patient's gait and balance. Most of these instruments have little role in a family physician's office as they are time-consuming and difficult to perform. The most useful of these tools is the "Get Up and Go" test. This is a simple office evaluation that involves asking the patient to arise from sitting, walk across the room or down the hallway, turn around, and return to his or her seat. During this test the following should be observed in the patient:

- Getting up from a chair and sitting down
- Bending over
- Stability of standing—ability to withstand slightest push
- Neck movement
- Initiation of ambulation
- Use of legs and feet
- Ambulation symmetry
- Ability to turn
- Need for balance support

If there is any suspicion of a potential gait disorder, a thorough gait evaluation should be conducted by a physical therapist. This assessment should include the role of assistive devices for improving the patient's gait and balance.
Other assessments may include the following:

- Routine sensory, proprioceptive (position and vibratory sensation), and cerebellar testing—To determine the possibility of neuropathies as contributing factors in a fall

- Cardiac exam—Note rate or rhythm disturbances
- Foot abnormalities—Such as callouses, ingrown toenails, metatarsal irregularities
- Mental status changes—Administer the Mini-Mental Status Exam (Appendix)
- The presence of rigidity or tremor—Observe hands at rest, test for rigidity by supinating/pronating wrist or flexing/extending elbow
- Vision and hearing—Visual changes associated with aging alone (decline in depth perception, poor dark adaptation, and presbycusis), as well as with diseases (cataracts, macular degeneration, and retinal tears/detachments), can alter perception of environment, making a fall more likely. Hearing is important in gait: listening to changes in flooring surfaces, appreciating obstacles, and adding to the central nervous system perception of each step.

A full functional assessment should be performed, including an evaluation of physical, cognitive, and functional abilities. Activities of daily living and instrumental activities of daily living should be documented.

DIAGNOSTIC TESTS

The evaluation of a patient with falls involves a thorough assessment of the surrounding events of the falls. Unlike dementia, in which a "standardized" set of laboratory tests should be performed on each patient, no set of recommendations has been developed for falls. In fact, research shows that falling is more a harbinger of frailty, and no battery of tests can be performed to determine the underlying cause of the falls.

- It is rare to find abnormalities in the blood or with radiographs that implicate specific causes for falls.
- Most physicians would consider performing chemistry panels, complete blood count, and urinalysis to assess for underlying illnesses.
- There is no role for routine electrocardiography, ambulatory cardiac monitoring, echocardiography, or cranial computed tomographic scans in individuals who fall. These tests are appropriate only if the history and physical exam indicate that there is a potential underlying disease that these tests could help elucidate.

WHEN TO REFER

Referral is rarely required in patients who fall, other than for the almost uniform involvement of physical and occupational therapists. The need for further clarification of the role of possible neurologic or cardiovascular causes is infrequent. Referral to an orthopedist should be considered in any patient who sustains a serious fracture.

TABLE 9.3. Management of Common, Treatable Causes of Falls

Diagnosis	Principle Findings	Management Strategies
INTRINSIC CAUSES		
Gait or balance disturbance	Abnormal "Get Up and Go" test Unstable Rhomberg Lower extremity weakness	Physical therapy evaluation and treatment Muscle-strengthening exercises Use of assistive devices
Arrhythmias	History of palpitations Abnormal cardiac exam Abnormal EKG and Holter monitor	Medications to control arrhythmias Cardiac pacemaker
CNS disorder (tumor, strokes, seizures)	History of syncope, seizure activity (urinary incontinence, tongue biting, loss of consciousness) Focal neurological findings	Antiplatelet therapy[a] Anticoagulation Antiseizure medications
Orthostatic hypotension	History of falling, dizziness, lightheadedness, syncope associated with standing or position changes	Alteration in medications Addition of mineralocorticoid
Vision or hearing deficits	Deficits on exam usually to moderate/severe levels	Evaluation and treatment of vision and hearing disorders if possible Use of assistive devices for stability Increased lighting
Acute illness (infection, acute cardiac ischemia or failure, acute GI bleed, rupture, obstruction)	Fever, tachycardia, pain Acute CNS change	Treat acute illness
Chronic disorders (dementia, Parkinson's disease, severe arthritis)	Evidence on history and physical of the disease process	Optimize therapy of the chronic illness Physical therapy evaluation and management Assistive devices
EXTRINSIC CAUSES		
Poor shoewear	Shoes with more than 1/2-inch heels Slippers or sandals	Solid-soled shoes Canvas running shoes
Fall in bathroom	Lack of grab bars, shower seats, wet flooring	Handyman to install grab bars and shower seats Nonslip floor coverings

continued

TABLE 9.3. *continued*

Diagnosis	Principle Findings	Management Strategies
Fall on stairs	Stair steps uneven, chipped, loose Railings/banisters inadequate or loose Poor lighting	Evaluation and repair of stairs Improve lighting around stairs Change housing to single level
Poor furniture, loose carpeting or flooring, slippery rugs	Furniture low to the ground or easily tipped over Rug backing not adherent Carpeting loose at edges	Remove furniture, rugs Repair carpeting Secure flooring
Poor lighting	Inadequate light in hallways, stairwells, living areas (bulbs less than 100 watts)	Increase lighting; may need new electrical wiring

^aAnticoagulation with warfarin needs to be reevaluated, as the risk of its use increases in fallers.

TABLE 9.4.   Additional Management Efforts to Reduce Risk of Fall

Evaluate household for potential risks
Have patient record characteristics and circumstances of all falls
Improve lighting at home
Instruct patient in strengthening exercises
Instruct patient on moving, changing positions
Review important extrinsic factors
Set up method to obtain help if debilitating fall occurs
Use assistance devices if necessary (grips, shoes, walkers)

MANAGEMENT

After a complete history and physical exam the physician may be unsure of the exact cause of any specific fall. However, in most patients there is usually a combination of intrinsic and extrinsic factors that need to be addressed. Table 9.3 below summarizes the common causes of falls and their management. Table 9.4 lists general steps to help reduce the risk of falls.

PATIENT EDUCATION

A patient information sheet on preventing falls is included in the Appendix. The following are key points to convey to patients:

- As people get older, their risk of falling goes up.
- Unresolved health problems can contribute to the risk of falling.
- The risk of falling can be reduced by removing barriers and obstacles in the home and by using supports such as walkers, canes, and railings.
- Problems with vision, hearing, and/or feet can cause falls.
- Discuss medications with the doctor. Sometimes medicine can cause falls.
- Report any dizzy spells, feeling "light-headed," or falls.
- If dizziness occurs on standing or sitting, change positions more slowly.

FOLLOW-UP

The timing for follow-up of patients who have fallen depends on the presumed cause of the fall. In general, as noted above, most falls imply that the patient is becoming more frail and that close follow-up for impending problems will be indicated. Besides following up for acute treatments and safety recommendations, observation and intervention are important to monitor for the following:

- Nutritional problems
- Decrease in ability to perform activities of daily living
- Mental status changes
- Self-esteem issues
- General activity level
- Depression

SUGGESTED READINGS

Rubenstein LZ, Robbins AS, Josephson KR, et al. The value of assessing falls in an elderly population: a randomized clinical trial. Ann Intern Med 1990;113:308-316.

Steinweg KK. The changing approach to falls in the elderly. Am Fam Phys 1997; 56:1815-1822.

Tinetti ME, Baker DI, McAvay G, et al. A multifactorial intervention to reduce the risk of falling among elderly people living in the community. N Engl J Med 1994;331:821-827.

Tinetti ME, Williams CS. Falls, injuries due to falls, and the risk of admission to a nursing home. N Engl J Med 1997;337:1279-1284.

CHAPTER 10

"Comfort Care" for Terminal Illness

The family physician will be called on to manage many patients with illnesses that are expected to cause death in a relatively short time, usually defined as a further life expectancy of 6 to 12 months. Death is not a preventable outcome and should not be viewed as a treatment failure. The tragedy of modern medical care is the lack of active management of the dying process.

The family physician must have the medical knowledge and skills necessary to provide for all the needs of the terminally ill. This has been named "comfort care" and must be applied with as much vigor and skill as any type of curative care. Comfort care should be planned and skillfully implemented by the physician when the situation dictates its timely application.

Comfort care focuses on control of symptoms, patient comfort, and maintenance of function. The family, as well as the patient, must be involved in comfort-care plans. The concerns in the care of the terminally ill include psychosocial and medical issues. Much of what is therapeutic in comfort care can be accomplished by the presence of a caring physician. The overall approach can be summarized in three points:

- Be prepared for problems.
- Be sensitive.
- Be there.

The overall goal is to allow the patient a dignified, relatively pain-free, meaningful death—a peaceful death—accepted and not feared, not accompanied by intolerable pain and suffering, and surrounded by loved ones.

In addition, the approach to terminally ill patients requires a knowledge of the following:

- Ethical issues
- Medical decision-making standards
- Hospice programs
- Grieving
- Bereavement

CHIEF COMPLAINTS

The following symptoms typically affect individuals with terminal illnesses, irrespective of their specific disease process:

• Pain
• Anxiety
• Dyspnea
• Constipation
• Nausea
• Urinary retention
• Anorexia and poor nutrition

Pain Presentations

Frequent and accurate pain assessment is the foundation of good pain control. A physician's judgment of the patient's pain is an inadequate method of assessment. Studies have demonstrated that physicians frequently underestimate pain severity. The most effective mechanism is to ask the patient how much pain he or she is having. The standard approach uses a quantitative pain scale, usually a 1-to-10 ranking, where 1 is no pain and 10 is the worst pain the patient has ever experienced. Some other options are as follows:

1. Have the patient draw a vertical line on a horizontal line scale:

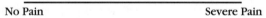

No Pain   Severe Pain

2. Have patient circle a face on a happy face–to–sad face scale

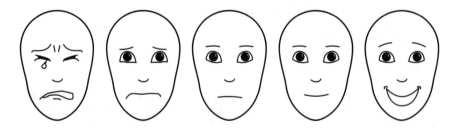

In cognitively impaired or noncommunicative patients, pain assessment is more difficult. In these cases most experts recommend assessing the patient's physical signs:

• Tachycardia
• Agitation
• Facial grimacing
• Verbalization such as moans and groans

Pain is the result of, or can be aggravated by, other factors. In the treatment of pain the following aggravating conditions must be addressed:

• Anxiety
• Depression
• Fear
• Fatigue
• Loneliness
• Inflammation
• Immobilization

Anxiety/Agitation

The dying process is consistently associated with anxiety. Anxiety can come from physical conditions such as pain or dyspnea, or from psychosocial issues such as loneliness or fear. Anxiety manifestations include apprehensiveness, hypervigilance, pain, agitation, anger, and depression. There are no quantitative measures for anxiety, and the patient's perceptions cannot always be used as the gold standard. In dying patients it is reasonable to assume the universal presence of anxiety and always address it in the therapeutic plan. A certain amount of "existential anxiety" is legitimate in the dying patient, but pathologic anxiety occurs when the intensity is so overwhelming as to interfere with effective functioning in life.

Chronic medication use and alcohol abuse can contribute to anxiety-like symptoms. Agitation, often accompanied by sweating, tremors, and fears of doom, can be the extreme manifestation of anxiety, or it can be a manifestation of delirium or dementia.

Dyspnea

Shortness of breath or alterations in breathing patterns usually indicate hypoxia, but may result from other symptoms associated with dying such as pain or psychologic states. The assessment of a terminally ill patient with dyspnea includes a physical evaluation looking for signs of congestive heart failure, pneumonia, or noncardiopulmonary disease. Blood measurements of oxygenation, hemoglobin, and renal function are important. A chest x-ray and an electrocardiogram (EKG) may be helpful. These tests may be unnecessary if the etiology is obvious or if the patient is near death and the focus of care is simply comfort and the rapid relief of symptoms.

Constipation

Constipation is universal in patients on narcotics or at bed rest and is common in most patients with a terminal diagnosis. The presentations of constipation can be stool related such as firm or infrequent bowel movements or can be more nonspecific such as the following:

- Abdominal pain
- Bloating
- Nausea
- Urinary incontinence
- Urinary retention

There is no quantitative measure of the occurrence or severity of constipation. Most patients report that a formed bowel movement every 48 to 72 hours is "natural." Caregivers for bed-bound patients usually attempt to achieve a semisoft stool every 24 to 48 hours. A good history and physical exam are the best ways to evaluate a patient for constipation. A rectal exam will help determine the presence of a potential fecal impaction.

Nausea and Vomiting

Nausea is a bothersome and uncomfortable symptom that is frequent in patients with terminal illnesses. There is no quantitative measure to assess nausea, and it can vary rapidly in intensity. Nausea is commonly the result of medication, constipation, new gastric irritation, or the underlying disease process itself.

Vomiting in terminally ill patients is extremely unpleasant and can increase pain and anxiety. It may be a transient nuisance or a persistent, obnoxious problem. Persistent vomiting is usually the result of one of four causes:

- Medications
- Gastrointestinal (GI) obstruction
- Brain metastasis
- Metabolic abnormalities
  - Diabetic ketoacidosis
  - Uremia
  - Hypercalcemia

Assessment of nausea and vomiting requires a review of medications and a physical evaluation, looking for gastrointestinal or central-nervous-system illness. Potential tests include serum chemistry panel, computed tomographic scan, and barium upper gastrointestinal studies.

Urinary Retention

Most terminally ill patients will have urinary retention at some point during their care. It can occur at any time during a terminal illness, but is most common when patients are forced into an immobile state. Urinary retention can result from obstruction by an enlarged prostate or from impacted stool. Bladder atony caused by neurologic impairment or intrinsic bladder disease can cause retention.

Urinary incontinence and painful or decreased urinary output may be indicators of urinary retention. A physical exam may detect a distended bladder or a prostatic or impacted stool obstruction. A urethral catheter will relieve the obstruction, and further workup can follow as indicated.

Patients with urinary retention have a high incidence of urinary tract infections and are commonly plagued with uncomfortable bladder spasms and overflow incontinence.

Anorexia and Poor Nutrition

Eating issues occur frequently in terminally ill patients. They commonly present as a lack of interest in eating or a lack of appetite or as comments that food does not taste good. Patients with nausea may become anorectic. Malnutrition is common—some patients will have frank cachexia. Eating issues may result from reactions to medication, poor-fitting dentures, esophageal infections or dysmotility, gastric irritation, or tumor-related problems.

HISTORY AND PHYSICAL EXAMINATION

The initial database necessary to care for a terminally ill patient begins with a standard history and physical examination focusing on the underlying disease state. A complete list of current medications is needed. A focus on the current symptoms is important, and it is essential to review these symptoms at each visit.

DIAGNOSTIC TESTS

When the focus is on comfort and function and not unnecessarily on prolonging the dying process, it is important to evaluate whether a particular diagnostic test is in fact necessary or whether it would be another irritant to the patient. In fact, it often better to avoid drawing blood and obtaining an imaging procedure rather than to cause unnecessary pain and suffering. The periodic measurement of the patient's hemoglobin/hematocrit electrolytes, serum drug levels, or prothrombin times are usually without benefit. There is no role for measuring any serum tumor marker in patients who are terminally ill.

GENERAL MANAGEMENT ISSUES

Treatment is always based on the goal of maximizing comfort and function. Decisions should be discussed and the potential consequences of options understood. Every decision to intervene should be weighed in terms of its altering the road to death that the patient will take. Continuing chronic medications or using new drugs or therapies should be evaluated for their benefit in providing comfort to the patient. Should the patient continue on antidiabetic agents, antiarrhythmic agents, anticoagulants? Should antibiotics ever be used, or should new medications be started to treat steroid-induced hyperglycemia or tumor-induced deep venous thrombosis? Is there any role for invasive procedures in providing comfort care? Each of these questions needs to be carefully evaluated in the management of a terminally ill patient.

Some decisions may be made early in the course of the terminal condition that will still impact on the patient's course to death. A classic example is the decision to place a nephrostomy tube in a patient with ureteral obstruction from a cervical cancer. The decision to drain the urinary system will prevent a uremic death, but has the potential to increase the chances of more pain from the advancement of the cancer. There are no hard and fast rules for the physician to follow with these decisions. The physician and patient need to discuss each, honestly weighing the benefits in terms of prolonging quality life and maximizing the options for a comfortable death. The sin of modern medical care is the prolongation of the dying process because of lack of attention to management issues.

The principles of comfort care must be adapted to be helpful to each patient. Most patients need this expertise as they approach their death. Some patients with terminal illnesses will want to pursue a curative medical approach up until the last breath. For others, a full hospice-style approach will best meet their needs. For many, the situation lies somewhere in between— wanting to pursue some therapies to cure the disease or to somewhat lengthen life such as chemotherapy, hormonal therapies, or parenteral nutrition, but not wanting further hospitalizations or other, more invasive, painful, or frightening therapies.

Patients with terminal illnesses will progress through fairly typical phases:

- Phase 1: The patient is ambulatory, eating, and death seems far away.
- Phase 2: The patient experiences progressive disability, usually with the gradual loss of independence in various areas of the activities of daily living such as dressing, eating, ambulating, toileting, and hygiene.
- Phase 3: The patient spends days to weeks confined to bed.

The role of psychosocial support cannot be overemphasized. The physician should support and facilitate psychosocial interventions from any and all who can benefit the patient such as social workers, clergy, family, and friends. The dying process is a time when many relationship issues are discussed, when old wounds can be healed, or when final love can be expressed. The physician should facilitate the preparation of the family for the loss of their loved one. Wills, funeral plans, and aiding the survivors' grieving can be handled during this time.

Crucial elements of the initial and ongoing management of a patient with a terminal illness include a discussion of the following:

1. Future goals and personal values
2. Establishment of a mutually understood plan for supported hydration and feeding

3. Advanced planning: completion of an advanced directive such as a living will or a durable, medical power of attorney

Future Goals and Personal Values

Each patient will be at a different place in his or her understanding of the disease and anticipation of the dying process. The family physician should directly ask about the patient's understanding of his or her condition and concerns about future care with questions such as: "Can you share with me your fears and concerns?" "What are your specific worries?" and "How can we best manage your condition together?"

It is important for the physician to assist the patient with the following:

- Encourage the patient to talk about fears and desires.
- Be clear in stating up front your commitment to the patient and to the goal of maximizing comfort and function and minimizing pain and suffering.
- Work with the patient to identify family members' roles in the patient's care; many terminally ill patients will spend part if not all of their last months at home with family caregivers.

Artificial Hydration and Feedings

At some point in the process of caring for a terminally ill patient, the physician should address artificial hydration and feedings. Artificial hydration and feedings are defined as any modality used to get food and water into the patient other than through the patient's mouth. This includes any type of tube or intravenous feedings, as well as intravenous hydration. Patients and families are best served if a clarification of these issues can be accomplished before the need arises. Some facts surrounding these topics include the following:

- Medical and legal standards are clear that artificial hydration and feeding are like any other medical intervention—open for discussion about whether they should be used.
- There is no evidence that patients experience more pain or suffering if they die without food or water. In fact, death from overhydration is unpleasant.
- Food and water can prolong life; however, this may be considered an undesirable prolongation of the dying process.

Advanced Planning

An advanced directive is a statement of the patient's desire for future care. It is an essential part of care for terminally ill patients and, for that matter, all patients. The advanced directive is usually a written statement, although an oral statement can be legally accepted.

Two common formats are recognized in every state: the living will and the durable power of attorney for health care (DPAHC). These type of forms are available in every state, usually through the state medical associations or from the state department of health. A patient information sheet on advanced directives is included in the Appendix.

A living will is a document that allows a patient to state his or her wishes regarding the use of medical interventions that could potentially prolong his or her life. Living wills vary by state. Some states use forms with prewritten statements that can be checked off by patients. Others are less structured and allow patients to write in their wishes. Living wills usually allow for patients to comment on the use of cardiopulmonary resuscitation, extraordinary medical intervention, artificial hydration and feedings, pain management, and other issues important to the patient. Living wills commonly discuss initiation, continuation, withholding, or withdrawing conditions of these therapies.

The fundamental use of the DPAHC is to ensure that an individual is assigned to make health-care decisions for the patient in the event that the patient is unable to make his or her own decisions. The assigned individual may be a friend or family member, but not a health-care provider involved in the patient's care, and is known as the patient's agent, proxy, or surrogate. DPAHCs may contain information similar to living wills. The patient is best served if his or her agent and physician are aware of the patient's desires. There is no requirement for an attorney to complete these documents, but witnesses are usually required.

Predicting Course of Terminal Illness

One of the most difficult aspects of caring for a patient with a potential terminal illness is predicting future disease course. Many diseases do not have a clear "terminal phase." For example, what symptoms or signs does a patient have with atherosclerotic cardiovascular disease, chronic obstructive pulmonary disease, or diabetes, indicating that they have 6 to 12 months to live? In many patients with cancer, the transition to a terminal phase may be at a time close to their death.

There are few guidelines in predicting the course for most illnesses. The best method is to do the following:

- Follow the patient closely.
- Listen to his or her needs.
- Evaluate his or her functional abilities.
- Be prepared to openly discuss the patient's disease state, its anticipated course, prognosis, and therapy options, including the option to enter into a comfort-care mode. In virtually all medical conditions there are staging or grading systems that allow the physician to determine the patient's progression from mild to moderate to severe disease states.
- Assess the patient's response to therapies and note when these therapies no longer appear able to control the manifestations of the disease state.

A frequently used method to assist physicians in determining a patient's prognosis is the Karnofsky Performance Scale (Table 10.1)—a functional scale

TABLE 10.1.   Karnofsky Performance Scale

Functional Level of Performance	Score
Normal; no complaints related to disease process	100
Minor signs and/or symptoms of disease; able to carry out normal activities	90
Clear signs and/or symptoms of disease; able to carry out normal activities	80
Cares for self (intact ADLs) but is limited in normal activities	70
Requires occasional assistance with self care (ADLs)	60
Requires assistance with self care (ADLs) and frequent medical care	50
Requires special care and assistance; disabled	40
Severely disabled; hospitalization an option	30
Death approaching without aggressive action	20
Moribund; rapid progression toward death	10
Dead	0

ADL, Activities of daily living.

A score of 50 or less is predictive of death within 3 months in 93% of patients, and within 6 months in 99% of patients. Higher scores are poorer at predicting survival, as many patients can show a rapid progression to death from higher scores.

HOSPICE

Hospice is a philosophical movement that strives to assist people in the dying process. Hospice can be a place where dying patients are cared for or can be a type of care provided to individuals at home or in a nursing-home setting.

The Medicare Certified Hospice Benefit (MCHB) can be elected by Medicare patients as an alternative to utilizing their Part A–Hospitalization Benefits. This concept has been so successful that almost all insurance carriers and health plans now offer a hospice benefit that is patterned after the MCHB. Hospice services include evaluation and care by a team of professionals such as registered nurses, social workers, clergy, home health aides, nutritionists, and hospice physicians.

The hospice team approach can aid the physician in managing all of the issues that face the patient and family in the dying process. In addition, the hospice is responsible for providing care for the patient and family throughout the patient's remaining life and provides bereavement care for the family after the death of their loved one.

that has been used for patients approaching a terminal phase or for those in a terminal phase to predict time of death. The scale has been researched and tested with many illnesses and shown to be accurate and reproducible.

WHEN TO REFER

Many resources are available to the physician and patient to assist in providing comfort care. Local hospice programs are available in all communities and should be used readily by physicians. Hospice care will have all necessary ancillary services available, including social services, spiritual counseling, legal counseling, and advanced medical support for pain and symptom management. Usually, hospice programs can provide the patient and physician with broad support during the patient's dying process.

SYMPTOM MANAGEMENT

The management of individual symptoms in terminally ill patients follows a general stepwise approach:

1. Assess the severity of the symptoms.
2. Evaluate for the underlying cause.
3. Address the social, emotional, and spiritual aspects of the symptom.
4. Discuss treatment options with the patient and family, and treat specifically for the cause or nonspecifically if the cause cannot be determined.
5. Use therapies designed as around-the-clock interventions for chronic symptoms and as-needed interventions for episodic symptoms.
6. Reevaluate the control of the symptom periodically.

Pain

The major focus of most dying patients is the avoidance of pain. No one wants to experience discomfort, and the fear of pain plagues all terminally ill patients. Inadequate treatment of pain reflected the state of medicine over the past 50 years and should not be accepted in current medical care. Although a pain-free state cannot always be achieved, it should be the goal. Controlling pain in terminally ill patients requires attention to the following:

- Potential etiology of the pain
- Use of nonpharmacologic methods
- Use of a number of medications

Pain in a terminally ill patient is not always the result of the primary disease process. Sources of the pain commonly include fracture induced by the disease, constipation, urinary retention, fear and anxiety, and neuropathies. Evaluating the complaint of pain and looking for the specific etiology often helps guide therapy.

Nonpharmacologic interventions are important adjuvants, as well as primary mechanisms, for controlling pain. Fear and anxiety will increase pain levels regardless of the primary cause of the pain. Control of fear and anxiety can be very beneficial and can be assisted by the following:

- Counseling
- Imagery
- Hypnosis
- Meditation
- Religious intervention
- Heat
- Massage
- Ultrasound
- Transcutaneous electrical nerve stimulation (TENS) units
- Acupuncture

Many physicians have access to these modalities in their local communities or by referral to physical/occupational therapy or to hospice programs.

Medication use to control pain has been researched extensively, and many recommendations exist regarding its appropriate use. In general, medications used for terminally ill patients are divided into two categories: analgesics and adjuvants.

Analgesics
Analgesic use should follow the World Health Organization (WHO) guidelines as detailed in the Agency for Health Care Policy and Research (AHCPR) Guidelines for the Management of Cancer Pain. The WHO adopted the ladder concept toward analgesic use (Fig. 10.1).The WHO emphasizes the following:

- Begin with nonnarcotic analgesics and progress to stronger medication as necessary to control the patient's pain.
- There are clear data to support the efficacy and ease of use of oral analgesics.
- Analgesics should be given on a timed basis and not on an as-needed basis.
- The standard is to give the patient a base dosage at a fixed time and to have available additional analgesic medication to use between doses if the pain worsens.
- If frequent, in-between doses are being administered, the fixed dose should be increased. Long-acting preparations of nonnarcotic and narcotic analgesics, which last for 8 to 12 hours, are available.

Addiction or tolerance concerns should never be an issue for pain management in terminally ill patients. The most commonly used medication to treat pain in terminally ill patients is morphine. Oral morphine is highly ef-

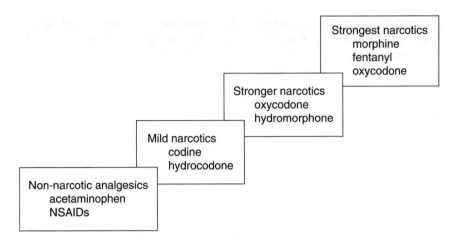

FIGURE 10.1. WHO ladder for pain control.

fective, easily administered in both long-acting and short-acting formulations, and is available in tablet, liquid, and parenteral delivery systems. Other narcotics are useful and can be used in patients who have problems with morphine therapy (Table 10.2). Meperidine (Demerol) is best avoided for pain control in terminally ill patients because there is an increased risk of seizures with chronic use.

Tramadol (Ultram) is a new, centrally acting, pain reliever used in both acute and chronic pain syndromes. Its exact mechanism of action is unknown. Maximum dose is 400 mg daily in divided doses (300 mg daily in divided doses for persons over age 75). It appears to have an analgesic effect similar to acetaminophen with codeine combinations (Table 10.3), with the major side effect of potentiation of seizure activity. Other side effects include nausea, dizziness, and gastrointestinal complaints. It should not be used in combination with an opioid preparation.

Adjuvants

Adjuvant therapy can be used in patients on narcotic analgesics (Table 10.4). Adjuvants are medications that act in concert with narcotics to decrease pain. These medications are nonnarcotics that either work through their own mechanisms to relieve pain or potentiate the effects of the narcotics. Adjuvant drugs frequently reduce the dosage of narcotics necessary to control pain and improve some of the side effects of the narcotic analgesics.

The Agency for Health Care Policy and Research has prepared a useful guideline for pain management.

TABLE 10.2. Dose Equivalents for Opioid Analgesics in Opioid-Naive Adults

Drug	Approximate Equianalgesic Dose		Usual Starting Dose for Moderate-to-Severe Pain	
	Oral	Parenteral	Oral	Parenteral
Morphine	30 mg q 3–4 h (repeat around the clock dosing) 60 mg q 3–4 h (single dose or intermittent dosing)	10 mg q 3–4 h	30 mg q 3–4 h	10 mg q 3–4 h
Morphine, controlled-release (MS Contin, Oramorph)	90–120 mg q 12 h	N/A	90–120 mg q 12 h	N/A
Hydromorphone (Dilaudid)	7.5 q 3–4 h	1.5 mg q 3–4 h	6 mg q 3–4 h	1.5 mg q 3–4 h
Levorphanol (Levo-Dromoran)	4 mg q 6–8 h	2 mg q 6–8 h	4 mg q 6–8 h	2 mg q 6–8 h
Meperidne (Demerol)	300 mg q 2–3 h	100 mg q 3–4 h	N/R	100 mg q 3 h
Methadone (Dolophine, other)	20 mg q 6–8 h	10 mg q 6–8 h	20 mg q 6–8 h	10 mg q 6–8 h
Oxymorphone (Numorphan)	N/A	1 mg q 3–4 h	N/A	1 mg q 3–4 h

Adapted from Management of Cancer Pain: Quick Reference Guide for Clinicians. DHHS Publication AHCPR 94-0592.

q = every; N/A = not available.

Cautions:

Recommended doses do not apply for adult patients with body weight less than 50 kg.

Recommended doses do not apply to patients with renal or hepatic insufficiency or other conditions affecting drug metabolism and kinetics.

Morphine, hydromorphone, and oxymorphone. Rectal administration is an alternative route for patients unable to take oral medications.

Anxiety and Agitation

The etiology for anxiety and agitation in a patient should be sought. It may have a psychologic basis, or it may relate to physical cause such as a distended bladder, hypoxemia, or uncontrolled pain. The treatment of anxiety begins

TABLE 10.3. Dose Equivalents for Combination Opioid/Acetaminophen or Aspirin Preparations in Opioid Naive Adults

| Drug | Approximate Equianalgesic Dose | | Usual Starting Dose for Moderate-to-Severe Pain | |
	Oral	Parenteral	Oral	Parenteral
Codeine (with aspirin or acetaminophen)	180–200 mg q 3–4 h	130 mg q 3–4 h	60 mg q 3–4 h	60 mg q 2 h (IM/SC)
Hydrocodone (in Lorcet, Lortab, Vicodin, others)	30 mg q 3–4 h	N/A	10 mg q 3–4 h	N/A
Oxycodone (Roxicodone, also in Percocet, Percodan, Tyulox, others)	30 mg q 3–4 h	N/A	10 g 3–4 h	N/A

Adapted from Management of Cancer Pain. Quick Reference Guide for Clinicians. DHHS publication AHCPR 94-0592

q = every; N/A -= not available; NR = not recommended.

Cautions:

Recommended doses do not apply for adult patients with body weight less than 50 kg.

Recommended doses do not apply to patients with renal or hepatic insufficiency or other conditions affecting drug metabolism and kinetics.

with behavioral techniques. Anxiety can be reduced in many terminally ill patients by providing an opportunity for the following:

• Discussion of their feelings and fears with a trained professional
• Formal counseling
• Prayer and meeting with a priest, pastor, or rabbi

The benefits of nonpharmacologic interventions in anxious or mildly agitated patients should never be underestimated.

Virtually all terminally ill patients will benefit from the use of mild anxiolytics (Table 10.5) such as benzodiazepines. Antidepressants may also be helpful when indicated. Those patients with extreme anxiety and agitation may need therapy with the major tranquilizers (Table 10.6).

Benzodiazapines as a group of drugs share common benefits and side effects. They are both sedative and anxiolytic They can accumulate in most patients and cause oversedation. Abrupt withdrawal in patients who have been taking them chronically can induce seizures. In the care of the terminally ill patients there is rarely difficulty because sedation and anxiolysis are the usual goal of therapy. Withdrawal of these drugs is not an issue in comfort care.

Buspirone (Buspar) is an anxiolytic belonging to the azapirone class. It can be effectively used to treat generalized anxiety disorders starting at 15 to 30 mg daily. Onset of therapeutic action occurs 1 to 2 weeks after initiation, and dosage should be limited to a maximum of 70 mg per day. There is no physical dependence nor are there withdrawal symptoms. The rare side effects include nausea, dizziness, headache, and nervousness.

TABLE 10.4. Adjuvant Medication

Adjuvant Medication	Mechanism of Action	Common Usage
STANDARD USE		
NSAIDs	Decrease inflammation Decrease pain	Added with any pain syndrome
Steroids	Decrease inflammation and edema	Added with bone pain or pain from metastatic disease; used with CNS tumors
Anxiolytics	Decrease anxiety	Added with any pain syndrome
Antidepressants	Affect CNS and PNS	Neuropathic pain and dysthymic mood
Psychostimulants	Stimulate CNS	Added when sedation from narcotics is a problem
Neuroleptics	Affect CNS	For sedation; decrease agitation
LIMITED USE		
Octreotide (Sandostatin)	Somatostatin analog	Muscle spasms; pain, limited use
Baclofen (Lioresal)	Muscle relaxant	Muscle spasms; spasticity
Chlorzoxazone (Parafon)	Muscle relaxant; sedative	Muscle spasms; spasticity
Cyclobenzaprine (Flexeril)	Muscle relaxant	Muscle spasms; spasticity
INVASIVE ADJUNCTS		
Radiation therapy	Decreases tumor size	Usually single bony metastasis
Beta-emitting agents	Decrease tumor size	Widespread metastatic disease
Intraspinal, intraventricular, intraforaminal injections	Injections of narcotics or local anesthetics causing nerve blockade, or direct action of narcotic	Pain in one dermatome, or intractable pain in lower body

TABLE 10.5. Commonly Used Anxiolytics

Agent	Approximate Dose Equivalents (mg)	Usual Range per 24 Hours (mg)	Half-Life (Hours)
LONG-ACTING[a]			
Diazepam (Valium)	5	5 to 60	20 to 100
Chlordiazepoxide (Librium)	10	15 to 100	5 to 30
Clorazepate (Azene, Tranxene)	7.5	15 to 60	30 to 200
Prazepam (Centrax, Verstran)	10	20 to 60	30 to 200
Flurazepam (Dalmane)	15	15 to 60	30 to 250
INTERMEDIATE-ACTING			
Halazepam (Paxipam)	20	40 to 160	14
Alprazolam (Xanax)	0.5	0.5 to 5	6 to 20
SHORT-ACTING			
Oxazepam (Serax)	15	15 to 120	5 to 15
Lorazepam (Ativan)	1	2 to 6	10 to 20
Temazepam[b] (Restoril)	10	10 to 30	10 to 20
ULTRASHORT-ACTING			
Triazolam[b] (Halcion)	0.25	0.25 to 1	1.5 to 4

[a]The longer duration of the long-acting drugs is the result of persistence of active metabolites.
[b]These drugs are marketed as hypnotics.

TABLE 10.6. Commonly Used Major Tranquilizers

Medication	Dosage (mg/day)	Potency	Sedation	Anticholinergic Effects	Side Effects
Haloperidol (Haldol)	0.5–10	High	+	+	Tardive dyskinesia; Parkinsonism
Riperidone (Risperdal)	0.25–3	High	+	0	Dyskinesias and hypotension
Thioridazine (Mellaril)	0–200	Low	+++	+++	Quinidine-like effects on the heart
Chlorpromazine (Thorazine)	10–100	Low	++++	+++	Hypotension and seizures
Clozapine (Clozaril)	12.5–200	Low	++	++	Agranulocytosis

+ = mild; ++++ = extreme.

TABLE 10.7. Antidepressants

Drug	Initial Dose (mg)	Usual Dose (mg)
SEROTONIN TRANSPORT INHIBITORS		
Fluoxetine (Prozac)	10 to 20	10 to 80
Fluvoxamine (Luvox)	25 to 50	100 to 300
Nefazodone (Serzone)	50 to 100	200 to 500
Paroxetine (Paxil)	10 to 20	20 to 50
Sertraline (Zoloft)	25 to 50	75 to 200
Venlafaxine (Effexor)	12.5 to 50	50 to 375
CYCLIC ANTIDEPRESSANTS		
Amitriptyline (Elavil)	10 to 50	150 to 300
Amoxapine (Asendin)	25 to 50	150 to 450
Clomipramine (Anafrinil)	25 to 50	150 to 250
Desipramine (Norpramin)	10 to 25	100 to 250
Doxepin (Sinequan, Adapin)	10 to 25	150 to 300
Imipramine (Tofranil)	10 to 50	150 to 300
Maprotiline (Ludiomil)	25 to 50	150 to 200
Nortriptyline (Pamelor)	10 to 25	75 to 125
Protriptyline (Vivactil)	5 to 10	15 to 60
Trimipramine (Surmontil)	25 to 50	150 to 300
MONOAMINE OXIDASE INHIBITORS		
Phenelzine (Nardil)	15	45 to 90
Tranycypromine (Parnate)	10	30 to 50
OTHERS		
Trazadone (Desyrel)	25 to 50	150 to 300
Buproprion (Wellbutrin)	75 to 100	300 to 450

Antidepressants can be used to provide relief of anxiety (Table 10.7). The tricyclic antidepressants are commonly used. In some studies selective serotonin reuptake inhibitors (SSRIs) are used.

The older tricyclic antidepressants have the side effects of cardiovascular problems (mostly orthostatic hypotension) and anticholingergic effects such as delirium, constipation, and urinary retention. The newer drugs, the selective inhibitors of serotonin reuptake and buproprion, may cause nausea, headache, or/and nervousness.

It is frequently difficult and sometimes impossible to find the right dose of the right drug to produce sufficient reduction in anxiety/agitation without oversedation. The best method for reducing anxiety/agitation without oversedation is to continue to try different drugs at various dosages.

Dyspnea

Dyspnea, or suffocation, is frightening. Relief of this sensation can be achieved by the following:

- Providing the patient with supplemental oxygen, even if the patient is not hypoxemic. In terminally ill patients it is unnecessary to perform blood gas measurements or oximetry prior to initiating oxygen.
- Circulating the air by opening windows and/or doors, and using a fan to provide air movement.
- Morphine is the drug of choice to treat dyspnea, and all dyspneic terminally ill patients should be given additional morphine to reduce the sensation of suffocation.

Constipation

Constipation is a difficult symptom to control and requires a vigilance equal to that for pain control. Treatment of constipation in patients on narcotics should be similar and as thorough as in patients not on narcotics. "The hand that writes the prescription for the narcotic should be the hand that writes the prescription for the laxative" is a common phrase heard at a hospice team meeting. Every terminally ill patient will need laxatives (Table 10.8). Where possible, patients should be encouraged to maintain basic, good bowel habits such as maintaining physical activity, drinking plenty of liquids, and eating specific foods such as fresh or dried fruits, vegetables, and foods high in soluble fibers such as grains, bran, nuts, and beans.

When the history or rectal exam reveals fecal impaction, the stool must be removed manually.

Nausea and Vomiting

The vast majority of terminally ill patients will experience nausea and vomiting caused by their underlying disease or medications. Gastric irritation should be identified and treated with antacids, H2 blockers, and sulcrafate (Carafate). GI obstruction should be ruled out and treated appropriately. Medications can be used alone or in combinations (Table 10.9). In many situations patients will require two or three medications to control their symptoms.

Urinary Retention

Urinary retention should be treated initially with drainage of the bladder with a urethral or suprapubic catheter. If the patient has a urethral obstruction secondary to a stricture or mass, there is a possibility of restoring normal voiding with treatment of these obstructions. However, atonic bladders usually require long-term catheter drainage.

The preferred method of long-term bladder drainage to reduce infection is self-intermittent catheterization rather than chronic, indwelling catheterization. However, in terminally ill patients who are approaching the time of their

TABLE 10.8. Drug Groups and Specific Medications for Treatment of Constipation

Drug Groups and Specific Medications	Common Doses	Comments
BULK AGENTS		
Methycellulose (Citrucel)	1–4 tbsp/day	Effective at 12–72 hours; inexpensive; side effects include gas, bloating
Psyllium (Metamucil, Konsyl)	1 tbsp qd–tid	
Barley malt extract (Maltsupex)	12–32 g bid	
Calcium polycarbophil (Fibercon)	1 tablet qd–qid	
LUBRICANTS		
Mineral oil	1–2 tbsp bid	Effective within 8 hours; distasteful to some; mild efficacy
OSMOTICS		
Lactulose (Cephulac, Chronulac)	2–4 tbsp, repeat q 4 hours prn	Effective at 4–8 hours; nonabsorbable; treats moderate to severe constipation; electrolyte imbalance with ricinoleic acid
Sorbitol (70%)	2–4 tbsp, repeat q 4 hours prn	
Ricinoleic acid (Castor Oil)	1–2 tsp as needed	
STIMULANTS		
Senna (Senokot)	1–2 tablets qd	Most effective; effect within 6–12 hrs, can induce GI cramping, dermatitis
Bisacodyl (Dulcolax)	5-mg tabs or 10-mg suppositories	

death, chronic use of Foley catheters is more practical and comfortable. Chronic, indwelling Foley use has been studied extensively in recent years, and there is fair consensus about appropriate care (Table 10.10).

Chronic-use catheters are important in all patients with lower body pressure ulcers. Patients without pressure ulcers who are bed-bound can use absorbent pads if preferred.

External collection devices, although available, are rarely if ever used in women and only occasionally in men because of the difficulty in ensuring urine containment.

In some situations death from sepsis may be seen as allowing a natural

TABLE 10.9. Medications Used to Treat Nausea and Vomiting

Medications	Dosage	Side Effects
PHENOTHIAZINES		
Prochlorperazine (Compazine); chlorpromazine (Thorazine)	5–10 mg PO or 25 mg PR bid–qid 10–100 mg PO	Anticholinergic; extrapyramidal reactions
BENZAMIDES		
Metoclopramide (Reglan); cisadpride (Propulsid)	5–10 mg PO qid 10 mg PO qid	Delirium; depression; extrapyramidal reactions
SEROTONIN ANTAGONISTS		
Ondansetron (trade) Droperidol (Inapsine)	8 mg PO qd or bid 0.5–2 mg IV or IM	Sedation

TABLE 10.10. Chronic Foley Catheter Care

- Foleys should be a closed-drainage system.
- Avoiding entry into that system is the most important factor in reducing the incidence of infections.
- The catheter should be changed monthly.
- No surveillance cultures should be done.
- There is no role for the use of prophylactic antibiotics to prevent infections.
- Infection of the urine should be treated only if fever, bladder spasms, or dysuria are present and only if the patient and physician agree that therapy is desired.

process to intervene. If treatment is pursued and the physician decides to obtain cultures, they should be obtained from a newly inserted catheter to ensure validity.

Anorexia and Poor Nutrition

A new onset of gastric irritation or a reaction to medication should be considered. However, the most common cause of anorexia is the impact of the disease on the patient's sense of hunger. All terminally ill patients will have some degree of malnutrition, some even frank cachexia. Patients with terminal illnesses may have poor nutrition from easily treatable conditions such as poor-fitting dentures and oral/esophageal candidiasis.

Every effort should be made to preserve and encourage oral hydration and nutrition. The evaluation should give consideration to oral, dental, and esophageal issues.

Anorexia from gastric irritation or obstruction may be treated and adequate oral intake returned. The vast majority of patients will not have these issues and will have anorexia from their underlying disease or medications.

The use of appetite stimulants can benefit some patients. The most commonly used agent to improve interest in eating is megestrol acetate (Megace), in doses up to 800 mg/day. Other treatment options may include the following:

- Steroids
- Prednisone
- Dexamethasone
- Dronabinol (an FDA-approved tablet form of tetrahydrocannabinol)
- Metoclopramide (Reglan)
- Cyproheptadine (Periactin)

Doses are not clearly established or standardized for this indication. Patients can be started on lower doses and moved upward with the maximum being limited by real and potential side effects that affect the quality of life.

The patient who wishes to eat should be given food and water. Once a patient ceases drinking and eating, the caregivers should encourage, but not force, the intake of food or water. The roles of the following interventions should be clarified prior to the time they might be considered:

- Enteral tube feedings
- Gastrostomy tube placement
- Use of parenteral nutrition

As noted above, allowing a patient to die without artificial hydration or nutrition may be appropriate management of the near-death patient.

MANAGING THE LAST HOURS

The last hours or days of the dying process can be the most difficult for the patient, family, and physician. Fortunately for a vast majority of patients, the last hours or days are spent in a comatose state, which appears to be a comfortable death. However, for some the end can be a harrowing process. The patient can experience extreme agitation, dyspnea, and struggle between attempting to live and die. The following can be very beneficial in managing these situations:

- An extra dose of morphine
- An anxiolytic

This is not a dose calculated to end the patient's life but a minor increase designed to take away the fear and struggle of the process. There is a fine line here between physician-assisted death and ease of suffering that hinges on intent. The skillful management of death with the intention of comfort care does not support the willful taking of the patient's life.

Some patients can benefit from the use of anticholinergics to dry respiratory secretions. To alleviate the "death rattle" that some patients experience, the following can be very effective:

- Atropine or hyoscyamine drops
- Scopalamine patches

"It's okay to go," or a similar comforting statement by the family, clergy, or physician can allow a patient to die more quickly. There are many such almost spiritual, or "cosmic," events that surround the process of death. We may not understand them, but we should be open to them and work with the patient and their family to support a peaceful death.

FOLLOW-UP

The terminally ill patient will require close follow-up visits or phone calls to manage the dying process effectively. The patient's clinical condition and symptoms can change rapidly. It is important to give the patient and family a sense of control and management of the unpredictable process. Caregivers in the household should be reminded about the need to handle financial, funeral, and emotional issues in advance. "Being there" is the single most important aspect of the physician's role in managing the dying process. By reassuring the patient and family of one's constant attention to the details, they will come to understand the commitment that the physician shares in ensuring a peaceful death.

BEREAVEMENT

Much lay literature exists about grief and bereavement. Each person and family will grieve in their own way. The physician should provide emotional support through open communication and a sharing of the understanding of the loss that has been experienced. Hospices typically will have professionals who are well versed in the bereavement process and its management. There is a role for medical intervention for a family member if the grieving symptoms become overwhelming, commonly with anxiety or vegetative signs of depression.

SUGGESTED READINGS

Brody HM, Campbell ML, Faber-Langendoen, K. Withdrawing intensive life-sustaining treatment. Recommendations for compassionate clinical management. N Engl J Med 1997;36(9):652–657.

Levy M. Pharmacologic treatment of cancer pain. N Engl J Med 1996;335:1124–1132.

Marwick C. Geriatricians want better end-of-life care. JAMA 1997;277:445–446.

American Geriatric Society Clinical Practice Committee. Management of cancer pain in older patients. J Am Geriatr Soc 1997;45:1273–1276.

Patient Information: Living with Congestive Heart Failure

What is congestive heart failure (CHF)?

Despite how it sounds, the term "heart failure" simply means your heart is not pumping blood as well as it should. Heart failure *does not* mean your heart has stopped working. "Congestive" means fluid is building up in your body because your heart is not pumping correctly.

What causes CHF?

Any disease that affects the heart and interferes with the circulation can lead to heart failure. Some of the most common causes of CHF include the following:

- Coronary artery disease
- Heart attack
- Congenital heart disease
- Problems with the heart muscle
- High blood pressure
- Problems with heart valves
- Abnormal heart rhythm
- Toxic substances (such as alcohol abuse)

What are some of the symptoms of CHF?

Call your doctor if you have any of these symptoms, especially if you have had heart problems before.

- Shortness of breath when walking or climbing stairs
- Shortness of breath when lying flat
- Waking up breathless in the night
- Feeling tired or weak
- Swelling of the legs (usually feet or ankles)
- Swelling of the neck veins
- Rapid weight gain (1 or 2 pounds a day for 3 days in a row)
- Chronic cough

What tests will I have to check if I have CHF?

Your doctor will probably suspect CHF based on your medical history, your symptoms and a physical exam. He or she might also order some of the following tests:

- Blood tests
- Urine tests
- Chest x-ray
- Electrocardiogram (monitoring of your heartbeat; also called EKG or ECG)
- Echocardiography (sound waves are used to produce pictures of the heart)

What treatment will I need?

Much can be done to improve the heart's pumping ability and treat the symptoms of CHF, but CHF cannot be completely cured. An important element of treatment is taking care of the underlying problems such as high blood pressure. Treatment also includes lifestyle changes and medicine. Your doctor may recommend the following changes:

- Eat a healthy diet—you will probably need to reduce the amount of salt you eat and maybe make other changes in your diet.
- Avoid alcohol—you may have to drink less alcohol or stop drinking it completely.
- Lose weight—if you are overweight, your doctor will probably recommend that you shed some pounds.
- Exercise—your doctor will help you determine how much and what kind of exercise you can do.
- Smoking—If you smoke, you will need to quit.

Lifestyle changes can be difficult to make, so get help from your family. You may also find support by talking with other people who have similar heart problems. Your doctor can give you information about these support groups.

What medicines will I need to take?

Many different medicines are used to treat CHF. You may need more than one medicine, depending on your symptoms. It might take a while to find the best medicine for you and the best amount of it. You also may have to change medicines if you have side effects. The most common medicines used to treat CHF include the following:

- **ACE inhibitors.** ACE inhibitors help dilate (open) your arteries and lower your blood pressure, improving blood flow.
- **Diuretics.** Often called "water pills," diuretics make you urinate more often and help keep fluid from building up in your body. They can also decrease fluid that collects in your lungs, which helps you breathe easier.
- **Digoxin.** Also called digitalis, digoxin helps the heart pump better. It may be combined with other medicines.

- **Nitrates.** Used commonly to improve blood flow to the heart.
- **Others.** Beta blockers, calcium channel blockers, hydralazine.

When you are taking medicine for CHF, you will need to have blood tests to check your potassium level and kidney function. How often you need blood tests depends on the kind of medicine you take and how much you take. If you have any side effects or concerns, talk to your doctor. To get the most benefit from your medicine, it is important to take it on time and exactly as your doctor says.

How often will I need to see my doctor?

At first, you may need to be seen as often as once a week to check on how you are reacting to your medicine. Once your doctor has made sure your medicine is right for you and you are feeling better, you may need to be seen less often.

When should I call my doctor?

You should call your doctor if you are short of breath or have swelling in your ankles or feet. Your should also call if you gain 3 to 5 pounds in 1 or 2 days. (To keep track of your weight, weigh yourself each day when you get up in the morning after urinating but before you eat anything.) You should also call your doctor if you have any questions about your condition or about your medicine.

American Academy of Family Physicians
The doctors who specialize in you

This handout was developed by the American Academy of Family Physicians in cooperation with the American Heart Association (1998 American Academy of Family Physicians, 8880 Ward Parkway, Kansas City, MO 64114-2797, http://www.aafp.org). Permission is granted to photocopy this material for nonprofit educational uses. Written permission is required for all other uses, including electronic uses.

FOR MORE INFORMATION

- American Heart Association: 800-AHA-USA1 (800-242-8721)
- National Heart, Lung, and Blood Institute Information Center: 301-251-1222
- Agency for Health Care Policy and Research: 800-358-9295 (Ask for "Living with heart disease: Is it heart failure?" publication no. 94-0614)

This handout provides a general overview on the topic and may not apply to everyone.
To find out if this handout applies to you and to get more information on this subject, talk to your family doctor.

Patient Information: Advance Directives and Do Not Resuscitate Orders

What is an advance directive?

An advance directive tells your doctor what kind of care you would like to have if you become unable to make medical decisions. When you are admitted to the hospital, the hospital staff will talk to you about advance directives.

Advance directives can take many forms. Laws about advance directives vary from state to state. You should be aware of your state laws regarding the scope and requirements that apply to advance directives.

A good advance directive describes the kind of treatment you would want to receive for different levels of illness. For example, the directives would describe what kind of care you want if you have a critical illness, a terminal illness or permanent unconsciousness. Advance directives usually tell your doctor that you do not want certain kinds of treatment when you are this ill. However, they can also say that you want a certain treatment, no matter how ill you are.

What is a living will?

A living will is one type of advance directive. It only comes into effect when you are terminally ill. Being terminally ill generally means that you have less than 6 months to live. In a living will, you can describe the kind of treatment you want in certain situations. A living will does not let you select someone to make decisions for you.

What is a durable power of attorney for health care?

A durable power of attorney (DPA) for health care is like a living will, but it becomes active any time you are unconscious or unable to make medical decisions. In a DPA, you select a family member or friend who will be your medical decision-maker if you become unconscious or unable to make medical decisions. A DPA is generally more useful than a living will. But a DPA may not be a good choice for you if you do not have another person you trust to make these decisions for you.

Living wills and DPAs are legal in most states. Even if they are not officially recognized by the law in your state, they can still guide your loved ones and doctor if you are unable to make decisions about your medical care. Ask your doctor, lawyer or state representative about the law in your state.

What is a do not resuscitate order?

A do not resuscitate (DNR) order is a request not to have cardiopulmonary resuscitation (CPR) if your heart stops or if you stop breathing (unless given other instructions, hospital staff will try to help all patients whose heart has stopped or who have stopped breathing). You can indicate with an advance directive form or by talking with your doctor that you do not want to be re-suscitated. In this case, a DNR order is put in your medical chart by your doctor. DNR orders are accepted by doctors and hospitals in all states.

Most patients who die in a hospital have had a DNR order written for them before they die. Patients who are not likely to benefit from CPR include people who have cancer that has spread, people whose kidneys do not work well, people who need a lot of help with daily activities, or people who have severe infections such as pneumonia that require hospitalization. If you already have one or more of these conditions, you should discuss your wishes about CPR with your doctor, either in the office or when you go to the hospital. It is best to do this early, before you are very sick and are considered unable to make your own decisions.

Should I have an advance directive?

Most advance directives are written by older or seriously ill patients. For example, a patient with terminal cancer might write that she does not want to be put on an artificial respirator if she stops breathing. This action can reduce her suffering, increase her peace of mind and increase her control over her death. You might want to consider writing an advance directive even if you are still in good health. An accident or serious illness can happen suddenly, and if you already have a signed advance directive, your wishes are more likely to be followed.

How can I write an advance directive?

You can write an advance directive in several ways:
• Use a form provided by your doctor.
• Write your wishes down by yourself.
• Call your state senator or state representative to get the right form.
• Call a lawyer.
• Use a computer software package for legal documents.

Advance directives and living wills do not have to be complicated legal documents. They can be short, simple statements about what you want done or not done if you cannot speak for yourself. Remember, anything you write by yourself or with a computer software package should follow your state laws. The orders should be notarized if possible, and a copy should be given to your family and your doctor.

 American Academy of Family Physicians
The doctors who specialize in you

This handout provides a general overview on the topic and may not apply to everyone.

To find out if this handout applies to you and to get more information on this subject, talk to your family doctor.

Patient Information: Caring for a Family Member with Dementia

Are behavior problems common in people with dementia?

Yes. Many patients with dementia—the name for an illness like Alzheimer's disease—have behavior problems such as shouting, agitation (being upset, frustrated and confused) and disturbed sleep. Wandering away and resisting care are other common problems. People with Alzheimer's disease may have strange thoughts, or they may imagine they hear or see things that are very upsetting to them (hallucinations).

Why do people with dementia become irritable and agitated?

The agitation can have many causes. Frustrating situations can cause people with dementia to become agitated. For example, a person with dementia may become agitated if he or she cannot get dressed, gives the wrong answer to a question or is challenged about his or her confusion or inability to do things. As a result, the person may cry, become irritable or try to hit, kick or hurt you in some way.

If the agitation has no obvious cause (such as a sudden change in surroundings or a frustrating situation), or if a person in your family becomes agitated very suddenly, he or she should be seen by a doctor. The sudden occurrence of agitation may be caused by infection, illness or injury, or by a medicine.

How can I deal with the agitation in my relative with dementia?

Even if the agitation is a chronic problem, there are ways of dealing with it. One of the most important things you can do is avoid situations in which your loved one might fail to remember something or forget to do something and become frustrated. You can try to have your loved one do the less difficult tasks. For example, instead of expecting your wife to get dressed all by herself, you can have her put on one thing by herself such as a jacket.

You can also try to limit the number of difficult situations the person must face. For example, showers can be taken every other day instead of every day. Also, you can schedule difficult activities for a time of day when your loved one tends to be less agitated. It is helpful to give frequent reassurance and avoid contradicting him or her.

What should I do if hallucinations are a problem?

If hallucinations are not making your loved one scared or anxious, you do not need to do anything. It is better not to confront people about hallucinations, because you will not be able to convince them that there are no voices or people, and arguing may just be upsetting.

If the hallucinations are scary, you can try to distract the person by getting him or her involved in a pleasant activity. If distracting the person does not work and the hallucinations continue, your doctor may want to prescribe some medicine to help. This medicine will not get rid of the hallucinations, but your loved one will be less upset by them.

What if my relative will not go to sleep at night?

First, try to make the person more aware of what time of day it is. You can have clocks placed where he or she can see them. You can keep curtains open so that he or she can tell when it is daytime and when it is nighttime.

Limit his or her consumption of chocolate, cola beverages, coffee and tea, since these substances contain caffeine and may keep him or her awake. Try to help your loved one get some exercise every day, and do not let him or her take too many naps during the day. Be certain that the bedroom is peaceful, since it is easier to sleep in a quiet room. If your family member has arthritis or another painful condition, ask your doctor if it is okay to give a medicine for pain right before bed, so pain will not interrupt sleep.

What if wandering becomes a problem?

Medicine usually does not help prevent wandering. Sometimes, however, very simple things can help with this problem. It is all right for your loved one to wander in a safe place such as in a fenced yard. By providing such a safe place, you may avoid a confrontation. If this does not work, a stop sign placed on the door or a piece of furniture placed in front of the door may remind your loved one not to go out that particular door. A ribbon tied across a door can serve as a similar reminder. Hiding the doorknob by placing a strip of cloth over it may also be helpful.

An alarm system (even just a few empty cans tied to a string on the doorknob) will alert you that your loved one is trying to leave a certain area. You might even have to place special locks on the doors, but be aware that such locks might be dangerous if a house fire occurs. Some people with dementia can open certain types of locks.

Where can I get more information?

The Alzheimer's Association provides support and assistance to people with dementia and their families. The Alzheimer's Association can be contacted by telephone, 800-621-0379, or by mail, 919 N. Michigan Ave., Suite 1000, Chicago, IL 60611-1676.

 American Academy of Family Physicians
The doctors who specialize in you

(1998 American Academy of Family Physicians, 8880 Ward Parkway, Kansas City, MO 64114-2797, http://www.aafp.org) Permission is granted to photocopy this material for nonprofit educational uses. Written permission is required for all other uses, including electronic uses.

A PPENDIX D

Folstein's Mini-Mental State Examination (MMSE)

MINI-MENTAL STATE EXAMINATION (MMSE)

Add points for each correct response.

	Score	Points
Orientation		
1. What is the:		
Year?	_____	1
Season?	_____	1
Date?	_____	1
Day?	_____	1
Month?	_____	1
2. Where are we?		
State?	_____	1
County?	_____	1
Town or city?	_____	1
Hospital?	_____	1
Floor?	_____	1
Registration		
3. Name three objects, taking 1 second to say each. Then ask the patient to repeat all three after you have said them. Give one point for each correct answer. Repeat the answers until patient learns all three.	_____	3
Attention and calculation		
4. Serial sevens. Give one point for each correct answer. Stop after five answers. Alternate: Spell WORLD backwards.	_____	5
Recall		
5. Ask for names of three objects learned in question 3. Give one point for each correct answer.	_____	3
Language		
6. Point to a pencil and a watch. Have the patient name as you point.	_____	2
7. Have the patient repeat "No ifs, ands, or buts."	_____	1
8. Have the patient follow a three-stage command: "Take a paper in your right hand. Fold the paper in half. Put the paper on the floor."	_____	3

9. Have the patient read and obey the following: "CLOSE
    YOUR EYES." (Write it in large letters.)   ____   1
10. Have the patient write a sentence of his or her choice.
    (The sentence should contain a subject and an object and
    should make sense. Ignore spelling errors when scoring.)   ____   1
11. Have the patient copy the design. (Give one point if all sides
    and angles are preserved and if the intersecting sides form
    a quadrangle.)   ____   11

                                                                      ____   = Total 30

In validation studies using a cut-off score of 23 or below, the MMSE has a
sensitivity of 87%, a specificity of 82%, a false positive ratio of 39.4%, and a
false negative of 4.7%. These ratios refer to the MMSE's capacity to accurately distinguish patients with clinically diagnosed dementia or delirium
from patients without these syndromes.
Source: Courtesy of Marshall Folstein, MD. Reprinted with permission.

For additional information on administration and scoring refer to the following references:

1. Anthony JC, LeReschel, Niaz U, et al. Limits of "Mini-Mental State" as a screening
    test for dementia and delirium among hospital patients. Psych Med 1982;12:
    397–408.

2. Folstein MF, Anthony JC, et al. Meaning of cognitive impairment in the elderly. J
    Am Geriatr Soc 1985;33(4):228–235.

3. Folstein MF, Folstein S, McHugh PR. Mini-Mental State: a practical method for
    grading the cognitive state of patients for the clinician. J Psych Res
    1975;12:189–198.

4. Spenser MP, Folstein MF. The Mini-Mental State Examination. In: Keller PA, Ritt
    LG, eds. Innovations in clinical practice: a source book. Vol 4. 1985; pp.
    305–310.

A

Patient Information: Living with Arthritis

What is arthritis?

Arthritis means inflammation of the joints. It causes pain and usually also limits movement of the joints that are affected. There are many kinds of arthritis. A type called osteoarthritis is the most common. Osteoarthritis is also called degenerative arthritis. But it does not usually cause severe crippling.

What causes osteoarthritis?

The exact cause is not known. A person may be at increased risk of osteoarthritis because it runs in the family. Osteoarthritis seems to be related to the wear and tear put on joints over the years in most people. But wear and tear does not by itself cause osteoarthritis. Osteoarthritis is not an inevitable result of aging or of wear and tear on the joint.

What happens when a joint is affected?

Normally, a smooth layer of cartilage acts as a pad between the bones of a joint. Cartilage helps the joint move easily and comfortably. In some people, the cartilage thins as the joints are used. This is the start of osteoarthritis. Over time, the cartilage wears away and the bones rub against one another.

The cartilage in people with osteoarthritis degenerates abnormally. As osteoarthritis gets worse, the breakdown of cartilage happens faster than the body can repair it. Bones may even start to grow too thick on the ends where they meet to make a joint, and bits of cartilage and bone may loosen and get in the way of movement. This can cause pain, joint swelling and stiffness.

Who gets osteoarthritis?

Osteoarthritis is more common in older people because they have been using their joints longer. Using the joints to do the same task over and over or simply using them over time can make osteoarthritis worse. Younger people can also get osteoarthritis. Athletes are at risk because they use their joints so much. People who have jobs that require the same movement over and over are also at risk.

Is there a treatment?

No cure for osteoarthritis has been found. But you do not have to become disabled. The right plan can help you stay active, protect your joints from damage, limit injury and control pain. Your doctor will help you create the right plan for you.

Will my arthritis get worse?

Osteoarthritis does tend to get worse over time. But you can do many things to help yourself. It is important to stay as active as possible. When joints hurt, people tend not to use them and the muscles get weak. This can cause contractures (stiff muscles), and you can lose your range of motion—it gets harder to get around. This causes more pain and the cycle begins again. Ask your doctor to discuss pain control with you, so that you can stay active and avoid this problem.

How arthritis will affect you also depends on your total health. For example, being too heavy means your joints have to carry extra weight. This can make osteoarthritis get worse faster and bother you more. This is especially true for arthritis of weight-bearing joints—like your hips, knees, or spine. Losing weight could lessen your symptoms if you are overweight.

Will medicine help?

Medicine you can buy without a prescription that reduces inflammation—such as acetaminophen (Tylenol), ibuprofen (Advil, Motrin, Nuprin, etc.), ketoprofen (Actron, Orudis), or naproxen (Aleve)—can help you feel better.

Medicine should be used smartly. You only need the amount that makes you feel good enough to keep moving. Using too much medicine may cause side effects. If you often take medicine that does not require a prescription, your doctor may give you a prescription medicine that can be taken less often to relieve pain. Talk to your family doctor about what

TIPS ON STAYING ACTIVE

- Lose weight if you are overweight.
- Exercise regularly for short periods.
- Go to a physical therapist if you can.
- Use canes and other special devices to protect your joints.
- Avoid lifting heavy things.
- Avoid overusing your joints.
- Do not pull on objects to move them—push them instead.
- Take your medicine the way your doctor suggests.
- Use heat and/or cold to reduce pain or stiffness.

is right for you. Watch out for false "cures" that may be advertised in magazines or newspapers.

Are special devices really helpful?

Yes. Special devices have been designed to help people with arthritis stay independent for as long as possible. These devices help protect your joints and keep you moving. For example, if you learn to use a cane the right way, you can help reduce the amount of pressure your weight puts on your hip joint when you walk by up to 60%.

Will exercise really help?

Exercise keeps your muscles strong and helps keep you flexible. This will also help you stay independent. But do not overdo it. Exercise in small amounts throughout the day with rest time in between. This will help you avoid injury and pain by not trying to do too much at once.

Exercises that do not strain your joints are best. This may include tightening your muscles and then relaxing them a number of times. You can do this with all of your major muscles several times throughout the day.

Another good exercise for arthritis is movement in a swimming pool, with much of your body's weight held up by the water. You may find this type of "aquacise" program available through a local YMCA, YWCA or other pool in your community.

Ask your family doctor what programs are available in your area. He or she may also suggest that you see a physical therapist to get you started.

SPECIAL DEVICES FOR PEOPLE WITH ARTHRITIS

- Canes
- Walkers
- Splints
- Shoe inserts or wedges
- Cushioned pads for shoes
- Nonslip soles on shoes (for traction)
- Special fasteners (such as Velcro) on clothing
- Large grips for tools and utensils (wrap foam or fabric around items with narrow handles such as pens)
- Lightweight appliances—those made from aluminum or plastic rather than glass
- Wall-mounted jar openers
- Electric appliances such as can openers and knives
- Mobile shower heads
- Bath seats
- Grab bars for the bathtub

Should I use heat or cold to ease pain?

Using heat or cold may reduce your pain and stiffness. Heat can be applied through warm baths, hot towels, hot water bottles or heating pads. Ice packs can also be used to help make you feel better.

Try alternating heat with ice packs. Some people find that using heat before activity and cold after activity is useful. Try different combinations and see what works best for you.

For more information on arthritis, call the Arthritis Foundation at 800-283-7800 or visit their Web site at http://www.arthritis.org.

 American Academy of Family Physicians
The doctors who specialize in you

A PPENDIX F

....

Patient Information: Understanding Parkinson's Disease

What causes the tremor of Parkinson's disease?

People with Parkinson's disease have a progressive loss of function of the nerve cells in the part of the brain that controls muscle movement. Tremors occur as a result of damage to the nerve cells.

The tremor, or "shakiness," of Parkinson's disease gets worse when the person is at rest and better when the person moves. The tremor may affect one side of the body more than the other, and can affect the lower jaw, arms and legs. Handwriting may also look "shaky" and smaller than usual. Other symptoms of Parkinson's disease include nightmares, depression, excess saliva, difficulty turning over in bed and buttoning clothes or cutting food, and problems with walking.

How is Parkinson's disease diagnosed?

No blood tests can detect Parkinson's disease. Some kinds of x-rays can help your doctor make sure nothing else is causing your symptoms, but x-rays cannot show whether a person has Parkinson's disease. The symptoms mentioned above suggest to a doctor that a person might have Parkinson's disease. If the symptoms go away or get better when the person takes a medicine called levodopa, it is fairly certain that the person has Parkinson's disease.

What causes Parkinson's disease?

In general, doctors do not know what causes Parkinson's disease. Some medicines can cause or worsen symptoms of Parkinson's disease.

Can medicines treat Parkinson's disease?

There is no cure for Parkinson's disease. However, medicines can help control the symptoms of the disease. Your doctor will discuss with you which medicines might help you.

Where can I get more information about Parkinson's disease?
Information is available from the following organizations:

American Parkinson's Disease Association, Inc.
1250 Hylan Blvd., Suite 4B
Staten Island, NY 10305
Telephone: 800-223-2732

National Parkinson's Foundation
1501 N.W. 9th Ave., Bob Hope Road
Miami, FL 33136-1494
Telephone: 800-327-4545

Parkinson's Disease Foundation
710 W. 168th St.
New York, NY 10032
Telephone: 800-457-6676

United Parkinson's Foundation and International Tremor Foundation
833 W. Washington Blvd.
Chicago, IL 60607
Telephone: 312-733-1893

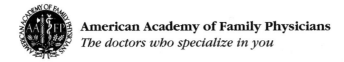 **American Academy of Family Physicians**
The doctors who specialize in you

This information provides a general overview on this topic and may not apply to everyone.
Talk to your family doctor to find out if this information applies to you and to get more information on this subject.

APPENDIX G

....

Patient Information: Urinary Incontinence: Embarrassing but Treatable

What is urinary incontinence?

Urinary incontinence means that you cannot always control when you urinate. As a result, you wet your clothes. This can be embarrassing. But it can be treated.

About 12 million adults in the United States have urinary incontinence. It is most common in women over 50 years old. But it can also affect younger people, especially women who have just given birth.

Be sure to talk to your doctor if you have this problem. If you hide your incontinence, you risk getting rashes, sores, and skin and urinary tract infections. Also, you may find yourself avoiding friends and family because of fears about your urine leaking and creating a scene. This embarrassment and loneliness can be avoided.

What causes incontinence?

Half of the time, urinary incontinence is caused by a medical condition other than a bladder problem. At other times, it may be caused by weakened pelvic muscles or other things. See the box on the next page for a list of causes. There are three main types of urinary incontinence:

Stress incontinence is when urine leaks because of sudden pressure on your lower stomach muscles such as when you cough, sneeze, laugh, rise from a chair, lift something or exercise. Stress incontinence usually occurs when the pelvic muscles are weakened, sometimes by childbirth, or by prostate or other surgery. Stress incontinence is common in women.

Urge incontinence is when the need to urinate comes on too fast—before you can get to a toilet. Your body may only give you a warning of a few seconds to minutes before you urinate. Urge incontinence is most common in the elderly and may be a sign of an infection in your kidneys or bladder.

Overflow incontinence is when you have a constant dripping of urine. It is caused by an overfilled bladder. You may feel like you cannot empty your bladder all the way and you may strain when urinating. This often occurs in men and can be caused by something blocking the urinary flow such as an enlarged prostate gland or tumor. Diabetes or certain medicines may also cause the problem.

CAUSES OF URINARY INCONTINENCE

- For women, thinning and drying of the skin in your vagina or urethra (the tiny tube that empties the bladder when you urinate), especially after menopause
- For men, oversized prostate gland or prostate surgery
- Weakened pelvic muscles
- Certain medicines
- Being confused or unsure of your surroundings
- Buildup of stool in your bowels
- Not being able to move around
- Urinary tract infection
- Problems such as diabetes or high calcium levels in your blood

Is urinary incontinence just part of growing older?

No. But changes with age can reduce how much urine your bladder can hold. Aging can make your stream of urine weaker and can cause you to feel the urge to urinate more often. This does not mean you'll have urinary incontinence just because you are aging. With treatment, it can be controlled or cured.

How can it be treated?

If your urinary incontinence is caused by something that can be treated, the incontinence will go away when the cause is successfully treated.

Incontinence can also be treated with special exercises, called Kegel exercises (see the box on the next page). These exercises help strengthen the muscles that control the bladder. They can be done anywhere, any time. You probably will not see a big difference for about 3 to 6 months after starting the exercises.

Women may experience better sexual response as a result of these exercises. Although designed for women, the Kegel exercises can also help men.

You can also train your bladder. Start by urinating at set intervals such as every 30 minutes to 2 hours—whether you feel the need to go or not. Then gradually lengthen the time between when you urinate—say by 30 minutes—until you are urinating every 3 or 4 hours.

You can practice relaxation techniques when you feel the urge to urinate before your time is up. Breathe slowly and deeply. Think about your breathing until the urge goes away. You can also do Kegel exercises if they help control your urge.

After the urge passes, wait 5 minutes and then go to the bathroom even if you do not feel you need to go. If you do not go, you might not be able to control your next urge. When it is easy to wait 5 minutes after an urge, begin waiting 10 minutes. Bladder training may take 3 to 12 weeks.

Losing weight if you are heavy may also help.

KEGEL EXERCISES

- To locate the right muscles, try stopping or slowing your urine flow without using your stomach, leg or buttock muscles. Another method is to pretend as if you are trying not to pass gas. When you are able to slow or stop the stream of urine, you have located the right muscles.
- Squeeze your muscles. Hold for a count of 10. Relax for a count of 10.
- Do this 20 times, three to four times a day.
- You may need to start slower, perhaps squeezing and relaxing your muscles for 4 seconds each and doing this 10 times a set three or four times a day. You can work your way up from there. Talk to your doctor about the best plan for you.

Biofeedback has also been used to overcome incontinence. Biofeedback uses complex machines that give pictures and sounds to show how well you are controlling your pelvic muscles.

Will medicine or surgery help?

Sometimes medicine helps some types of urinary incontinence. For example, estrogen cream to put in the vagina can be helpful after menopause for some women who have mild stress incontinence.

Several different kinds of surgery may be useful. Surgery is usually done to treat urinary incontinence only after other things have not worked or if the incontinence is severe.

American Academy of Family Physicians
The doctors who specialize in you

A *Patient Information: Decreasing Your Risk of Falls*

Who is at risk of falling?

Anyone can fall. The risk increases with age. Each year, falls occur in about one-third of people 75 years of age or older who are living in their homes. This increased risk of falling may be the result of changes that come with aging plus other medical conditions such as arthritis, cataracts or hip surgery.

What can I do to decrease my risk of falling?

Because most falls (75 percent) occur in the home, you should make sure your home is safe by following these tips:

- Make sure that you have good lighting in your home. As your eyes age, less light reaches the back of the eyes where your vision is located. The lighting in your home must be bright so you can avoid tripping over objects that are not easy to see. You should put night lights in your bedroom, hall and bathroom.
- Rugs should be firmly fastened to the floor or have nonskid backing. Loose ends should be tacked down.
- Electrical cords should not be lying on the floor in walking areas.
- Put hand rails in your bathroom for bath, shower and toilet use.
- Do not use stairs without rails on both sides for support. Be sure the stairs are well lit.
- In the kitchen, make sure items are within easy reach. Do not store things too high or too low. Then you will not have to use a stepladder or a stool to stand on.
- Wear shoes with firm nonskid, nonfriction soles. Avoid wearing loose-fitting slippers that could cause you to trip.

What else can I do?

Take good care of your body. Try to stay healthy by following these tips:

- See your eye doctor once a year. Cataracts and other eye diseases can cause you to fall if you do not see well.
- Take good care of your feet. If you have pain in your feet or if you have large, thick nails and corns, you should have your doctor look at your feet.
- Talk to your doctor about any side effects you may have with your medicines. Problems caused by side effects from medicine are a common

cause of falls. The more medicines you take, the more you risk having side effects from them, which raises your risk of falling.

- See your doctor if you have dizzy spells.
- If your doctor suggests that you use a cane or a walker to help you walk, please use it. This will give you extra stability when walking and will help you avoid a bad fall.
- When you get out of bed in the morning or at night to use the bathroom, sit on the side of the bed for a few minutes before standing up. Your blood pressure takes some time to adjust when you sit up. It may be too low if you get up quickly. This can make you dizzy, and you might lose your balance and fall.

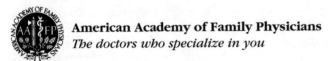

American Academy of Family Physicians
The doctors who specialize in you

(1998 American Academy of Family Physicians, 8880 Ward Parkway, Kansas City, MO 64114-2797, http://www.aafp.org) Permission is granted to photocopy this material for nonprofit educational uses. Written permission is required for all other uses, including electronic uses.

APPENDIX I

Patient Information: Hospice Care

What is hospice care, and what are its purposes?

Hospice is the name for a special program of care for terminally ill (dying) patients and their families. Rather than trying to cure an illness, hospice efforts are directed toward making the patient comfortable, easing pain and other troublesome symptoms, and supporting the family through a sad time.

The hospice care program tries to provide the best quality of life for dying persons by providing a holistic approach—that means giving spiritual, mental, emotional and physical comfort to the patients, their families and their other caregivers.

What is a hospice team?

The hospice team is a group of dedicated professionals, support staff and volunteers who understand the special goals of hospice care. The team includes doctors, nurses, social workers, chaplains, aides, and volunteers. The hospice team members focus their efforts on easing the symptoms of the terminally ill patient and providing support to the patient's family.

Is hospice care available to nursing home residents?

Yes. The services of hospice care programs are provided wherever patients are spending their final days, whether in their own home, in a family member's home or in a nursing home. The hospice team helps patients live out their final days with dignity and with as much physical comfort as possible.

The members of the hospice team try to help nursing home patients to be as free of pain as possible. They also try to help them be at peace with themselves and their illness. At the same time, the hospice team provides support, education and counseling to family members, nursing home staff and other nursing home residents who know the patient.

What specific services does a hospice program provide?

Hospice care programs can provide the following services:
- Nursing services with special expertise in symptom control.
- Training of family members in patient care, as appropriate.
- Spiritual and emotional support for both the patient and the family.

- Help with practical matters associated with terminal illness.
- Speech, occupational and physical therapies (when these services are considered useful by the hospice team).
- Coordination of services and care with the patient's family doctor.
- Through the Hospice Medicare Benefit, equipment and medicines (except a usual $5 copayment for each medicine) are paid for when they are ordered by the hospice team.
- Bereavement and support groups for families.
- Expert management of physical symptoms.

What is bereavement support?

Bereavement support is help in coping with the loss of a loved one. Grieving is a psychological process that nursing home staff members, family members and friends must go through when a person they love or take care of dies. It is necessary to feel the pain of grief in order to become whole again.

Normal grief has no timetable or calendar, and people experience grief in many different ways. Many people feel anger, loneliness, guilt, confusion and fear after a loved one dies. It helps to be able to talk about the person who has died.

Hospice is committed to helping people who are grieving. Hospice staff members and volunteers offer warm professional support to help family members with emotional healing and readjustment. Hospice respects the natural dying process and provides patients and family members with an opportunity for spiritual growth during this final phase of life.

 American Academy of Family Physicians
The doctors who specialize in you

This information provides a general overview on this topic and may not apply to everyone.

Talk to your family doctor to find out if this information applies to you and to get more information on this subject.

APPENDIX J
....

Annotated Bibliography

Cassel CK, Cohen HJ, Larson EB, et al. Geriatric medicine. New York: Springer-Verlag, 1997.

One of only a few authoritative and complete textbooks in geriatrics. Each chapter is thorough and readable. Has a number of useful tables, figures, pictures, and graphs. Some excellent chapters on ethics especially end of life care and value of achieving a peaceful death. Useful to have on your shelf, and it will come in handy for reading on a particular topic.

Hazzard WR, Bierman EL, Blass JP, et al., eds. Principles of geriatric medicine and gerontology. New York: McGraw-Hill, 1994.

Multiauthored text that covers the entire field of geriatrics in great depth and yet with clarity. The chapters on the geriatric syndromes are complete but wordy. The chapters on older adult internal medicine are excellent and each topic is well referenced. Not a book you will pick up to just read, but if you are looking for a fact, a great reference.

Kane RL, Ouslander JG, Abrass IB, eds., Essentials of clinical geriatrics. New York: Mc-Graw-Hill, 1994.

Excellent fundamental reference in geriatrics. Easy to read and complete in all the geriatric syndromes. Weakness is in the sections in older adult internal medicine. Outstanding figures, graphs, and tables. Perfect reference for the medical student and resident. Published as an inexpensive paperback text.

Reuben D, Yoshikawa T, Desdine RW, et al., eds. Geriatrics review syllabus. Dubuque, Iowa: Kendall/Hunt, 1996.

The definitive text on Geriatrics published by the American Geriatric Society. Authoritative core curriculum in Geriatric Medicine from which many geriatric exam questions are taken. Has its own test type questions with annotated answers and can be used for CME hours. Expensive because of the CME component. The best overall text for completeness. Each section is concise and easy to read.

Yoshikawa T, Cobbs E, Brummel-Smith K, et al., eds. Ambulatory geriatric care. St. Louis: Mosby–Year Book, 1993.

Paperback text that attempts to cover many topics in geriatrics, including the syndromes as well as topics, in Older Adult Internal Medicine. Each chapter is easy to read but occasionally incomplete. Some unique sections such as driving assessment and spiritual contributors to independence. I would recommend as an addition to your library but not as a primary text for the field.

173

Besdine R, Rubenstein L, et al., eds. Medical care of the nursing home resident. Philadelphia: American College of Physicians, 1996.

This book is a collection of articles written for the American College of Physicians by selected scholars in Geriatrics. The articles were to be a series in the Annals of Internal Medicine *but were compiled into this text. This text was distributed to graduate medical education programs nationally by the American College of Physicians. There are 4 sections covering the general approach to nursing home care, drug use in the nursing home, the common clinical conditions and some special considerations for nursing home patients. Each chapter is well referenced and there are many useful tables throughout the book. This is an excellent reference for teaching as well as practicing high quality nursing home care.*

United States Preventative Services Task Force, ed. Guide to clinical preventive services. Baltimore: Williams & Wilkins, 1996.

This is the second version of the United States Preventive Services Task Force (USPSTF) recommendations for clinical preventive services. The first edition, published in 1989, was a landmark reference for health maintenance. This edition is thoroughly updated and expanded. The topics cover recommendations for screening tests for early detection of diseases, immunizations to prevent infections, and counseling for risk reduction. This edition is heavily referenced with the available evidence to support or not support any given intervention. It is the gold standard text on preventive services.

Goldberg T, Chavin S. Preventive medicine and screening in older adults. J Am Geriatr Soc 1997;45:344-354.

A summary of the various recommendations for preventive medicine and screening in the elderly. Includes information from USPSTF 1996. A summary table is included that shows quality and grades of evidence.

Hoenig H, Nusbaum N, Brummel-Smith K, et al. Geriatric rehabilitation: state of the art. J Am Geriatr Soc 1997;45:1371-1381.

An excellent summary of the principles of geriatric rehabilitation. Specific disease rehab is included for strokes, cardiac diseases, deconditioning, hip fracture, and amputations. An essential reading for primary care physicians. An understanding of rehabilitation is essential in the care of the elderly.

Jahnigen DW, Schrier RW. Geriatric medicine. Cambridge, MA: Blackwell Scientific, 1996.

An excellent geriatric textbook with clearly written sections that are brief enough to be readable and yet thorough enough to be authoritative. The chapter on Parkinson's disease by Dr. L. Robbins is outstanding in its focus for the primary care physician. Dr. Robbins has lectured yearly for the AAFP on Parkinson's Disease and this chapter is an excellent example of his expertise. This text is well organized and referenced. An excellent addition for a family physician's office.

INDEX

Page numbers in *italics* denote figures. Those followed by a "t" denote tables.